Prevention of Head Injuries in Skiing

Prevention of Head Injuries in Skiing

Mechanisms, Experimental Study, and Prevention

Sooyoung Oh

Head of the Neurosurgery Section, Department of Surgery, Kantonsspital, Chur, Switzerland

174 figures and 13 tables, 1985

KARGER

Basel · München · Paris · London · New York · New Delhi · Singapore · Tokyo · Sydney

Cover illustration: © dpa, Deutsche Presse-Agentur GmbH, Frankfurt/Main

National Library of Medicine, Cataloging in Publication
Oh, Sooyoung
Prevention of head injuries in skiing: mechanisms, experimental study, and prevention / Sooyoung Oh
Basel; New York: Karger, 1985. –
Bibliography: p.
Includes index.
1. Athletic Injuries – prevention & control 2. Head Injuries – prevention & control 3. Skiing
I. Title
WE 706 036p
ISBN 3–8055–3978–9

Printed in Switzerland by Thür AG Offsetdruck, Pratteln
ISBN 3–8055–3978–9

Contents

Preface

Switzerland, a model country in so many ways, is also a model laboratory for studying injuries related to skiing. Though certainly not the only nation with a claim on Alpine terrain, Switzerland is more greatly dependent on the tourist industry than are France, Italy, Austria, and Germany. In certain Alpine areas of Switzerland, tourism may account for up to 80% of the economy. In this sense, snow is an important national resource, and skiing, apart from ranking as the nation's favorite sport, is an industry that has been cultivated with characteristic Swiss efficiency.

Not surprisingly, Swiss ski resorts are known for their superior facilities, lift equipment, and slope conditions as well as for their outstanding scenery and the famous personalities frequently photographed there. The country is thus ideally styled for an 'industrialized' recreational sport that depends on sophisticated personal equipment and well-organized transport installations, goes through fashions, and carries, as part of its popular appeal, an association of healthy physical exertion with an evening of relaxing in luxury.

In the past decade, these very attractions have created a serious problem in skiing because the number of serious and fatal head accidents linked to this sport has increased to an alarming degree in Switzerland itself and in every other country with facilities for downhill skiing.

This monograph, focused on head injuries and based on more than 10 years of experience in the Department of Neurosurgery at the Cantonal Hospital of Chur (Graubünden), documents the severity of accidents associated with skiing and explores their causes, covering both the obvious and some unexpected dangers of this sport.

For such a project, Switzerland has again served as a good model: the small geographic area of this country combined with its dense population of locals and tourists makes it possible for a neurosurgical department, such as ours, to gather experience and statistics on a sufficient scale to permit some generalizations.

As the record of cases seen and treated by us clearly shows, even the best and most immediate medical treatment of the head injuries is not always adequate to save the accident victim or prevent life-long handicaps. Head injuries in skiing are serious mostly, and increasing in frequency nowadays. It is for these reasons that strategies for prevention have been kept at the forefront of concern throughout this work.

Chur, January 1985 *S.O.*

1 Introduction

Brief Description of the Sport of Skiing

Downhill skiing is a sport based on the thrill of speed and the skill required to control it. The fascinating challenge of maneuvering under momentum has understandably determined the way in which the ski industry has utilized technology to make this popular sport even more attractive. Improvements in ski equipment and slope preparation technology have catered to the thrill of speed.

Though skiing as a mode of transportation dates back to antiquity, recreational skiing is a modern sport highly dependent on equipment. As in most sports, the technical capacity of ski equipment shows itself in the extreme case of competitive downhill racing, where speeds may reach up to 140 km/h. These televised races, held weekly throughout the season, are the ultimate association of skillful skiing with speed and the elegant beauty of human physiology responding to an extreme challenge of topography.

Despite its dependence on sophisticated and costly equipment, skiing remains the most anthropomorphic of sports where speed is given by the force of gravity. Though sports such as parachuting and hang gliding are also personal contests against the force of gravity, they differ from skiing in the sense that departure from the top of a slope is sailing over a landscape where the scale, though perceived at speed, is always human.

Yet the downhill skier's terrain is not a 'natural' one. It is an industrialized topography, populated with costly equipment, shaped and prepared to facilitate greater speeds, and, above all, cultivated to attract a profitable number of skiers. It has become an overcrowded landscape, and, for reasons to be described, a dangerous one (fig. 1/1).

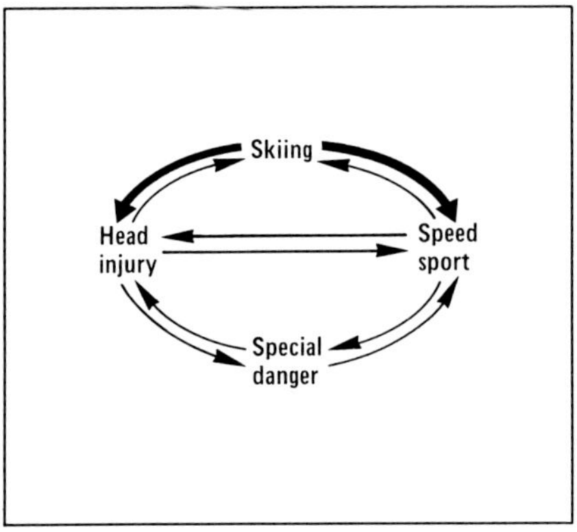

Fig. 1/1. Speed leads to head injuries.

The Risk of Accidents

All sports carry an accident risk, as do all activities involving speed [65]. In skiing, the manufacturing and marketing of lighter, faster skis has been paralleled by the safety-conscious improvement of boots and automatic bindings. As statistics show, these improvements have led to a marked reduction of leg and ankle injuries attributed to ski accidents [13]. On the negative side, the protection of legs and ankles has increased the risk to a far more vulnerable organ: the head (table 1/I).

The combination of higher skiing speeds with better boots and automatic bindings means that the skier involved in an accident no longer benefits from the natural 'brake' of skis that remain attached after a fall. Released from his skis, the accident victim flies, often headfirst. With the impact of a fall no longer absorbed by the lower limbs, the head becomes more susceptible to injury, and the number of fatalities associated with ski accidents increases.

Although comprehensive statistics are difficult to find, we do know that head injuries occurred in 4.5% of worldwide ski accidents in 1966 [64]. In figures from the Austrian Tyrol, the head was involved in 12.2% of the 6,034 injuries recorded for 1983 (table 1/I). These figures show an increase over those for 1981, where the head was involved in 10.7% of 3,225 total injuries [13]. Concerning leg injuries, these same figures showed a decrease from 59.5% in 1981 to 56% in 1983.

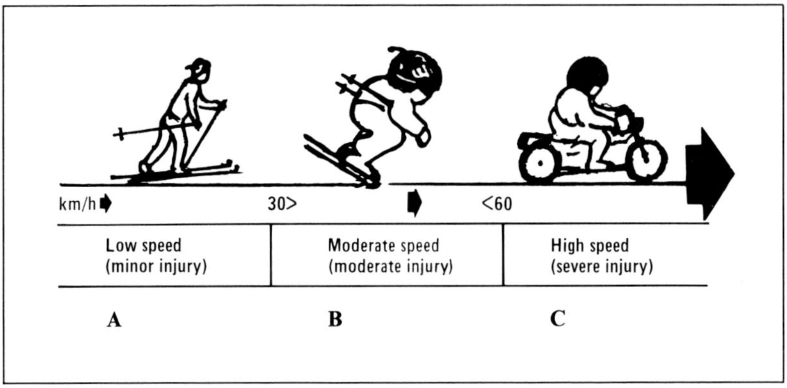

Fig. 1/2A-C. Speed coordinates to head injury.

Table 1/I. Increase in head injuries

	1981	1982	1983
Number of injuries	3,225	5,733	6,034
Legs, %	59.5	57.8	56.0
Head, %	10.6	11.9	*12.2*
Shoulder, %	2.3	11.3	11.4
Arm/hands, %	12.9	7.2	6.8
Others, %	14.7	11.8	13.6

This recent report of skiing accidents from the years 1981–1983 comes from the Tyrol, Austria.

In general, the risk of accidents in skiing correlates with speed in a way that is similar to risks in other forms of locomotion, such as bicycling or motorcycling, where the body of the victim is exposed. The injury of the human head and the speed (force) is coordinated absolutely (fig. 1/2): low speed to minor damage, high speed to severe injury. Cross-country skiing (fig. 1/2A) does not involve speeds of more than 30 km/h (low speed) and thus no head injuries have been yet reported. On the contrary, with speeds of more than 60 km/h (high speed) severe head injuries occur occasionally, as can be seen in motorcycle accidents, for example (fig. 1/2C). It is, however, obligatory for the motorcyclist to wear a crash helmet. Skiing (also cycling) involves moderate speeds (30–60 km/h), resulting in moderate injuries (fig. 1/2B). The moderate injuries mostly need medical care (with or without operation) and sometimes have posttraumatic sequelae.

It has also been observed that for accidents attributed to excessive, careless speed, males under the age of 25 account for the largest number of victims [39–41]. Furthermore, my observations show a higher incidence of head injuries during the month of February when the slopes are at their peak occupancy [41]. As would be expected, this crowded month is marked by the large number of severe and fatal accidents attributed to collisions between skiers (see fig. 2/3).

Yet, for the skier, slow speed is no guarantee of safety. Given the increasing likelihood that accidents will involve the head, coupled with the extreme vulnerability of that organ, serious skull fractures may occur at an impact speed of about 20 km/h (see fig. 2/1). The risk of head injuries is further complicated by the increasing number of skiers, which brings an increasing risk of collisions. In the case of collisions between slow and faster skiers, my observations indicate that it is most often the slower skier who suffers the more severe injuries (see fig. 3/9).

Pilot and Vehicle in One

The number of skiers grows steadily from year to year in parallel with improved access by transport and newly opened skiing areas, as well as improvements in skiing equipment [51]. With the improvement in equipment and preparation of the slopes, there is also an increase in speed which leads to an overall greater risk of accidents. High speed, uncontrolled skiing and high 'traffic density' on the slopes often result in very serious accidents. According to a private market research institute, even in 1967 there were about 1.4 million (now about 2 million) skiers in Switzerland [7] and about 50,000 skiing accidents annually [7]. According to the UN experts *Thierry, Quintina and La Mothe,* there were about 37 million skiers in the world in 1976, and by 1982 they were estimated to number about 55 million.

Every skier during the high season has witnessed 'traffic jams' at ski lifts and cable cars. Apart from the discomfort of having to wait, these traffic jams, and the overcrowding they represent, have an impact on accident risk that is best demonstrated by comparing the similarities and differences between car driving and skiing [41].

The similarities are self-evident. Both driving and skiing involve speed. Both take place on prepared and marked 'roads'. Both are open to the public, and both experience periods or seasons where traffic density is greater. Finally, both driving and skiing involve an accident risk directly related to the dual influences of speed and traffic density. As is the case with automobile accidents, most ski injuries can be attributed to either excessive or inadequate speed.

Here the similarities end abruptly and dramatically. Whereas driving, outside the extreme case of racing, is primarily a means of transportation, skiing is a sport dependent on the thrill of speed. On the slopes, every vehicular unit of skier and equipment has to be regarded as a sports model geared for speed and free to race without restraint. Second, no one needs a license to ski. Children and the elderly, healthy persons and semi-invalids, beginners and experts, the physically fit and the poorly conditioned can all depart down the slopes without having to pass a test of their qualifications to do so. Nor is travel across and down the slopes governed by traffic signals or safety regulations. There are no speed limits and no lanes for passing. Though slopes are marked according to degree of difficulty, no one controls who enters the 'expressways' where slow speed may be just as dangerous as excessive speed, and where a breakdown or fall may lead to serious collisions. Nor are the large number of children and young people who enjoy the thrill of speed but may lack the skill to control it, and who are frequently influenced by televised races to imitate a racing posture and cannonball carelessly down the slopes, controlled by regulations or even likely to be influenced by slope signs or warnings. In fact, the installation of a sign has little meaning for children and youngsters, as have street signs, unless they have been taught to obey them at home or in school.

Nor is the 'don't drive if you drink' maxim applicable to ski resorts. On the contrary, alcohol consumption, either with the noon meal, or often to excess as part of the evening relaxation, belongs to the culture of ski resorts, particularly in such wine-producing countries as France, Italy, Switzerland, Germany, and Austria.

Furthermore, skiing takes place on a one-way street, with all skiers moving from the top to the bottom of the slope (fig. 4/2). Though head-on collisions are only possible at crossings, the likelihood of collisions between slower and faster skiers increases in a one-way configuration where 'defensive' skiing is rendered virtually impossible for the slower, and often the more careful, skier. Nor is passing prohibited in areas of poor visibility. On the contrary, the courage to keep up speed around a dangerous blind curve,

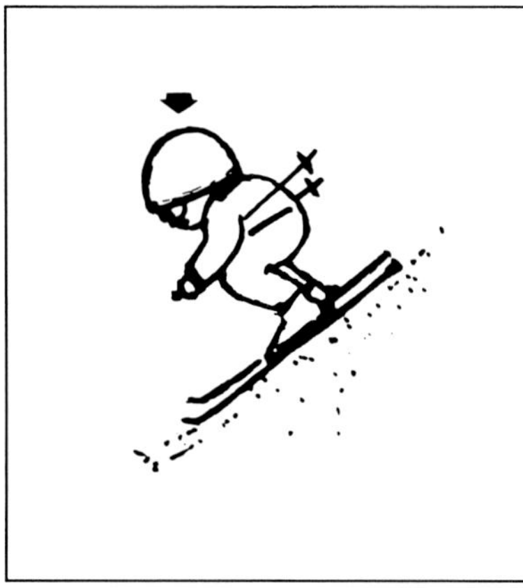

Fig. 1/3. The helmet protects life.

and then to rely upon skill and quick reactions to handle the 'surprise' situation, belongs to the suspense and appeal of this sport.

In terms of accident risk, perhaps the most important difference between the skier and the car driver rests in the fact that the skier is himself both pilot and vehicle in one. In this sense, the dangers shared by driving and skiing, seen against the striking dissimilarity of their safety regulations, become all the more ominous: the force that merely dents a fender can, when applied to the human head, produce a serious injury.

The following chapters describe ski accidents involving head injuries (especially for a 'typical type of head injury' namely the depressed skull fracture), examine the causes of these accidents, catalogue the outcome of treatment, and, above all, point out strategies for prevention. Since the skier is the vehicle as well as its pilot, preventive efforts must concentrate on reducing the risk of (accidents) while also making the vehicle itself more resistant to impact at its most vulnerable point. Otherwise, the increasing number of skiers and the resultant congestion on the slopes, the growing number of head injuries and the greater percentage involving the head will combine to form a trend where more and more splendidly healthy holidays on skis end in death or life-long handicaps. The simplest way of preventing head injuries in skiing is recommended here, namely the safety helmet (fig. 1/3).

2 The Causes of Accidents

Skiing at more than 20 km/h (fig. 2/1) may cause craniocerebral injuries [41]. Uncontrolled speed and carelessness lead to an increased risk of accidents while skiing [5, 6, 25, 39–42, 44, 46, 47]. The causes and types of head injuries are discussed and analyzed in this chapter.

Slope Accidents

The severity of head injuries mainly depends on the speed and slope conditions. Free fall accidents are divided into three categories: (1) minor fall (up to 30 km/h); (2) moderate fall (30–60 km/h), and (3) severe fall (over 60 km/h).

Free Fall

Accidents from Minor Falls

Depending on snow conditions, slight to severe head injuries will occur, hard or icy slopes being, of course, particularly dangerous. The application of force over a large area to the head (head hitting slope) usually causes closed brain injuries, with or without skull fractures (no depressed fractures), usually requiring conservative therapy. It is possible, but rare, for a chronic subdural hemorrhage to develop from light falls involving brain injury, and this has to be treated surgically. These light falls mostly resulted in concussion, which was usually treated conservatively in local hospitals or by us.

Over a period, increasingly severe headaches often occurred, and these were investigated by cerebral angiography (before CT was available) or CT when a slowly developing hemorrhage, such as a chronic subdural hematoma, was suspected.

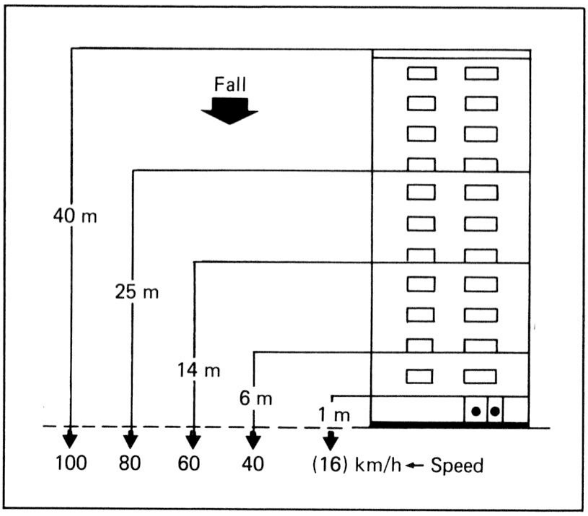

Fig. 2/1. Force of impact in relation to speed and to height of fall.

For example, a 42-year-old male (case 1) had had a minor fall on an open slope about 4 weeks before coming to our hospital. He went to a local hospital on the day of the accident, where slight brain contusion was found. He had since complained of minor headaches and 2 days before admission, he had sudden bitemporal headaches with dizziness and nausea. The pattern was of a typical chronic bilateral subdural hematoma (fig. 3/1). Surgery showed extensive chronic bilateral hemorrhage. His clinical condition was satisfactory after the operation, and he was discharged 3 weeks later symptom-free. A 54-year-old woman (case 2) had a minor fall while skiing on a soft slope 4 weeks previously. She suffered mild concussion. No medical care was sought. As time went on, she suffered from recurrent mild headaches at irregular intervals, and shortly before hospitalization she had difficulty in writing and found that she dropped things more often. On examination a hematoma was found (fig. 3/2) and removed surgically. After 4 weeks the patient was discharged, and 3 months later at an outpatient check-up she was completely free of any discomfort.

Accidents from Moderate Falls

On an open slope with powder snow, a fall at 30–60 km/h usually causes mild to severe concussions. On the other hand, an icy or hard snow slope is very dangerous compared with a soft powder snow slope; severe craniocerebral injury, such as brain contusion with or without skull fractures may then occur. Most of these accidents affect children or young people. The head injuries, usually ranging from contusion of the brain with skull fractures to basal fractures, mostly require some weeks of medical care in hospital. If complications occur, such as intracranial hemorrhage or infections, or convulsive seizure, surgical procedures or special treatment are necessary. Brain contusions are often accompanied by residual problems.

For example, a 26-year-old male (case 3) fell on an open hard snow slope and immediately lost consciousness. He had a convulsive seizure which led to a deep comatose state. He was transferred to our Neurological Department as an emergency case. Skull X-ray revealed a linear fracture in the right temporobasal region (fig. 3/3). After 3 weeks of conservative treatment, his condition was good. Another 24-year-old male patient (case 4) fell on a hard, icy ski slope and suffered brain contusion and fell unconscious immediately. After examination (fig. 3/4, 5), the patient underwent immediate surgery. The patient's condition postoperatively improved so much that he could be discharged without any symptoms about 4 weeks later. He since had a convulsive seizure necessitating continuous anticonvulsive treatment. A third example shows a 17-year-old male patient (case 5) who fell on an open slope due to losing his balance. He lost consciousness immediately and was admitted to us as an emergency. Brain contusion was diagnosed and the patient was treated conservatively. He was discharged 3 weeks later with a postcontusion syndrome. 3 years later, the patient suffered from continuous dull headaches and deterioration in memory. CT scan surprisingly revealed a serious communicating hydrocephalus aresorptiva (fig. 3/7). Surgery was then performed to construct a ventriculo-abdominal shunt. He no longer complains of headaches and his memory is better.

Accidents from Severe Falls

A fall on a hard slope at high speed causes severe head injuries, such as severe brain contusion with or without a brain stem lesion. This is usually accompanied by linear fractures of the skull (possibly with a basal fracture).

Jumps at high speed on any powder snow slope can cause serious brain and brain stem contusions, often with a fatal outcome, even after aggressive surgical treatment.

For example, the case of a 17-year-old male (case 6) who injured himself in an accident while jumping at high speed during skiing. After the accident, his consciousness became impaired and he rapidly became more somnolent. He was admitted to hospital as an emergency case in a deeply comatose condition. Neurological examination showed a midbrain syndrome. Despite aggressive surgical treatment, the patient died 2 days later following severe brain damage (fig. 3/8).

Discussion

As is obvious, speed and force are interconnected. Skiing involves speed. Slow skiing results in weak forces, while high-speed skiing produces strong forces. A force of more than 2 kN at ca. 20 km/h (fig. 2/1) causes head injuries, with various types of damage (to skull or brain or both) depending on the energies of impact.

High-speed skiing can lead to severe injuries and, of course, injuries from slow-speed skiing are less serious. The highest speed recorded in downhill races is over 140 km/h. High speed produces a pleasing sensation which is particularly attractive to children and young skiers [31]. However, it also involves great risk of accidents. I have classified 3 degrees of accidents from falls at 3 different speeds. The threshold of impinging forces causing severe head injuries is above 60 km/h, because of the histophysiological reactions of the components of the human skull and brain.

The blue powder snow slope provides an adequate skiing speed and is ideal for health and enjoyment. On the other hand, the black hard ski slope automatically produces higher speeds, which increase the danger of falls, for example. Jumping on the open slope is possible only at high speed, and then, when an accident occurs, severe head injuries usually result (case 6).

Good physical condition and the blue powder snow slope with an adequate skiing speed are ideal for health and avoidance of accidents and severe head injuries.

Collision with Another Skier

On many occasions innocent skiers have suffered severe head injuries in collisions caused by others skiing at speed and carelessly. The circumstances of these accidents are comparable with accidents to cars on the road, similar conditions and problems existing.

The following is a summary of our collision accidents in the last 8 years: 21 pairs involved in serious collisions (head to head) were treated (tables 2/I, 3/I), 15 patients surgically. The high number of accidents during

Table 2/I. Severe injuries, group a

Patient No./name		Age/sex	Injuries	Treatment
1	R.P.	18/M*	BC, EH, DF – right temporal	operation
2	A.O.	65/F	BC, DF – left frontal	operation
3	H.O.	9/M	BC, DF – left frontal	operation
4	K.A.	16/M	BC, CH – left frontal	operation
5	G.C.	22/F	BC+MBS, DF – right frontal	operation †
6	S.B.	17/F	BC, BF – right frontal	operation
7	H.O.	51/M	BC, SF – right temporal	operation
8	B.E.	22/M	BC, MBS	operation †
9	M.F.	23/M	BC, SF – right frontal	operation
10	S.A.	16/M	BC	conservative
11	C.B.	17/F	BC, BF – left frontal	operation
12	B.I.	11/F**	BC, MBS, DF – right occipital	operation †
13	K.D.	8/F	BC, BF – right frontal	conservative
14	C.P.	10/M	BC, liver injury (H)	operation
15	G.H.	17/M	BC, BF – right frontal	conservative
16	T.C.	22/F	BC, BF – right temporal	conservative
17	S.V.	36/F	BC, SF – right frontal	conservative
18	A.R.	47/M	BC, EH, SF – right parietal	operation †
19	S.H.	19/M	BC, SF – right parietal	operation
20	W.M.	28/F	BC	conservative †
21	K.J.	47/M***	BC, DF – right frontal	operation

* = Case 7; ** = case 8; *** = case 9.
BC = Brain contusion; EH = epidural hematoma; DF = depressed fracture; (H) = helmet worn; CH = cerebral hematoma; BF = basal fracture; MBS = midbrain syndrome; SF = skull fracture.

February is noteworthy (13 pairs) and the reason for this is the high 'traffic density' on the ski slopes during that month [52]. Severe head injuries were mostly suffered by children and young skiers, mainly male, who ski aggressively at high speed and carelessly.

It is interesting to note that, in collisions, one of the participants often suffers a severe head injury while the other receives only minor injuries, if any.

Of 21 severely injured in group a, 5 patients died from the brain damage. 11 patients with minor head injuries in group b were treated as outpatients. Unfortunately, I did not attend 5 of the partners in the collisions in

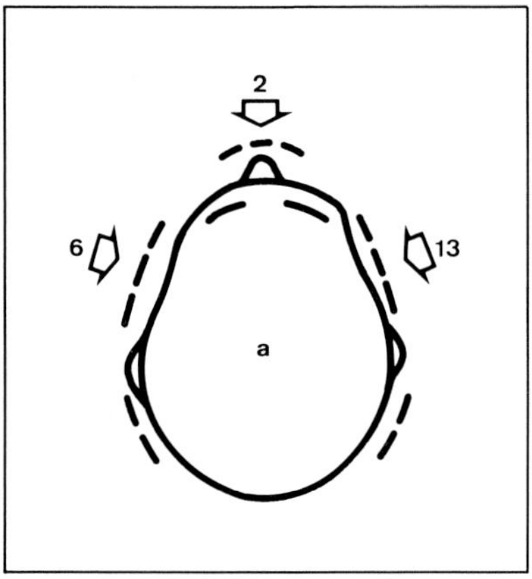

Fig. 2/2. Location of head injuries in group a.

group b. One child wore a safety helmet, no head injury resulting. It is noteworthy that all 16 known patients in group b had frontal injuries, whereas the 21 severely injured in group a mostly had parietotemporal injuries (fig. 2/2). 19 cases received parietotemporal injuries, 13 of these on the right.

An example of head to head collision is shown by case 7, an accident involving an 18-year-old and a 43-year-old male on an open slope (fig. 3/9). Both were knocked unconscious immediately. Whereas the older patient suffered a frontobasal skull fracture with slight brain contusion, the other received an extended, closed depressed fracture as well as severe brain contusions. The 43-year-old man was treated for 2 weeks conservatively and was discharged symptom-free. The 18-year-old man was rushed to hospital by helicopter where emergency surgery was performed (fig. 3/10, 12). Although the postoperative course was good, he was discharged 3 weeks later still suffering from posttraumatic complaints such as occasional headache and dizziness.

Another accident occurred between a 14-year-old boy and an 11-year-old girl (case 8). The girl fell on the ski slope and fractured her leg. She could not get up and stayed where she was on the slope. Shortly afterwards, the boy collided with the girl who was on the ground hitting her head at full speed (fig. 2/3). Despite aggressive surgery, the girl died 2 days later due to cardiac and circulatory arrest as a result of severe brain injury (fig. 3/14).

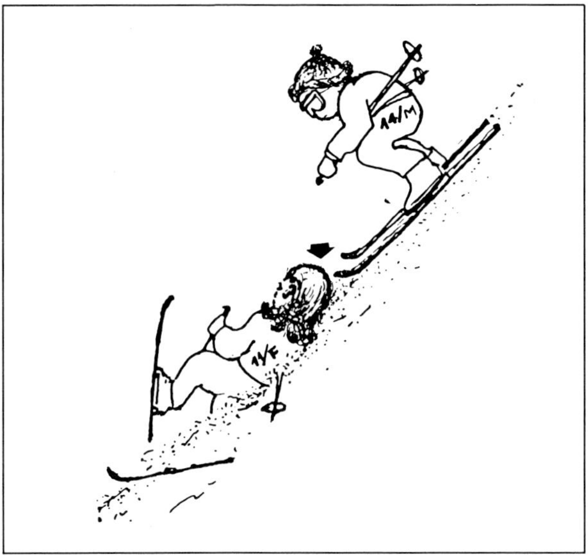

Fig. 2/3. Circumstance of accident.

A third example is that of a 46-year-old male (case 9) who was skiing carefully and slowly on an open slope when a young man ran into him at high speed. Both patients were admitted together as emergencies. The young man suffered a slight brain contusion and was discharged without any symptoms after 9 days of conservative treatment. However, the 46-year-old man had received a severe open head injury and surgery was performed immediately (fig. 3/17, 18).

Discussion

Collision accidents resulting in severe head injuries are increasing in frequency [41].

The data on the patients in the last 8 years have been collated and the types of injuries have been analyzed. The first noteworthy point is the discrepancy in the severity of the injuries that the two collision victims suffer. In the group of those slightly injured (b), only frontal injuries occurred, whereas the patients in the group with severe injuries (a) mostly suffered skull fractures and brain damage in the temporoparietal area. This is primarily due, of course, to the inherently stronger frontal bone as compared with the parietotemporal region of the skull (fig. 4/20).

An analysis of this study shows that those in group a were slower skiers than those in group b. This indicates that b crashed into a, and thus b is guilty (at fault). This is also supported by the fact that 75% of group b were men as compared with 55% men in group a. 77% in group b were under 18 years of age versus 62% in group a.

As all skiers move downhill on the slope, frontofrontal collisions are normally impossible, in contrast to road accidents. The only frontofrontal collisions took place at ski slope crossings, for which reason all crossings of ski slopes should be eliminated or made safe by means of overpasses. Most collisions take the form of a slower skier being run into from the side or behind by a faster skier. This accounts for the inequality in severity, one suffering a severe injury of the lateral region of the head and the other only a slight lesion of the frontal area.

Contrary to the common belief that slow speed results in safe skiing, an analysis shows that it is the lower skier who suffers more severe injuries. Furthermore, collision of adult skiers with children (especially small children) accounts for most injuries to children, because they are weaker than adults. For example: on March 2, 1984, a 3-year-old girl skier suffered a head injury in a collision with an adult on the open ski slope. The girl skier suffered a closed depressed fracture of the left parietal region (fig. 2/4) with epidural hematoma, which underwent immediate surgery.

On the basis of these considerations, one arrives at the conclusion that 3 factors are important for ski collisions: (1) high density of skiers on the slopes, which will probably increase further in future, especially in February; (2) excessive speed and uncontrolled skiing, the case usually being that the slower or weaker skier has to suffer for the carelessness of others, and (3) those severely injured are not usually at fault.

Injury Caused by Ski Equipment

In a free fall on the slope, quite often head injuries that are caused by one's own equipment or that of another skier occur; almost always objects of small surface area are involved, and these usually lead to depressed fractures. These injuries are often caused by faulty adjustment of the automatic ski binding which, in a fall, opens immediately or, even without opening, projects the ski (ski-tip) against the head (fig. 2/5).

A case in which the ski was involved was that of a 24-year-old male (case 10) who fell on an open slope and the tip of his ski struck his head. He

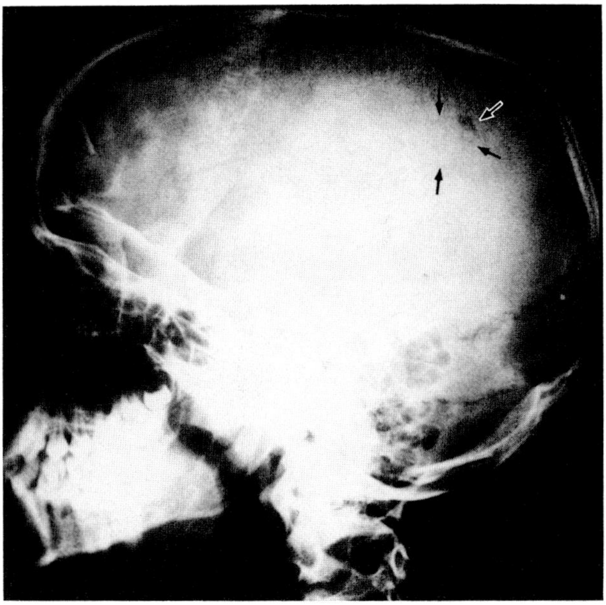

Fig. 2/4. 3-year-old skier suffered closed depressed fracture from collision with adult.

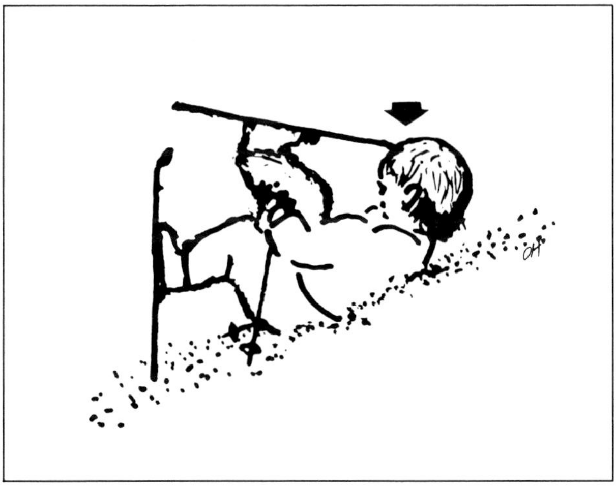

Fig. 2/5. Fall with tip of own ski striking the head, usually resulting in a depressed fracture.

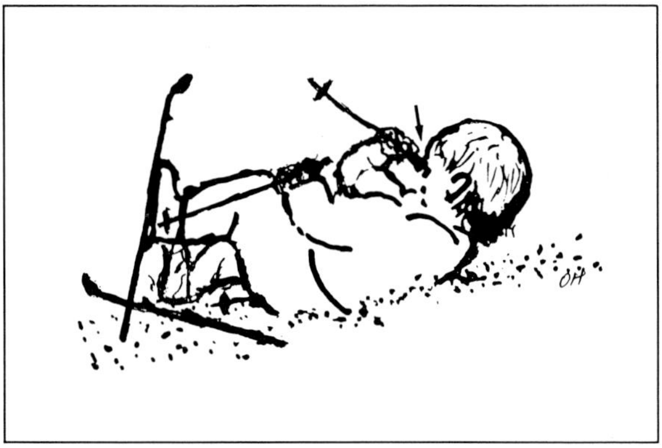

Fig. 2/6. Fall and blow against eye from own ski stick.

suffered brief amnesia. This resulted in an open depressed fracture of the skull which required immediate surgery. He was discharged 12 days after operation so that he could return to his home in Germany. Collision with ski equipment often involves accidents with ski sticks. The parts injured range from the thumb to the entire body. A serious eye injury was caused by a skier's own stick (case 11, 37-year-old male). The patient fell while skiing and the handle of the ski stick hit his right eye (fig. 2/6). He was transferred to us as an emergency. Enucleation of the right eye had to be performed (fig. 3/20). Another patient (case 12) fell on the open slope and the sharp end of the ski stick hit his forehead. The 15-year-old boy lost consciousness briefly. Immediate first aid by rescuers was given. When he was admitted to hospital, it was decided to perform surgery immediately (fig. 3/21). No complications arose in the postoperative course, and the patient was discharged 2 weeks later.

Slipping or Sliding

Slipping and sliding accidents can be very serious. Careless skiing during snowfall or fog on the slopes often cause these types of accidents, especially to children and young skiers. Usually, extensive cerebral contusion, with or without linear skull fracture (or basal fracture), results, while depressed fractures are rare. Other injuries are mostly to the chest and abdomen, and leg fractures.

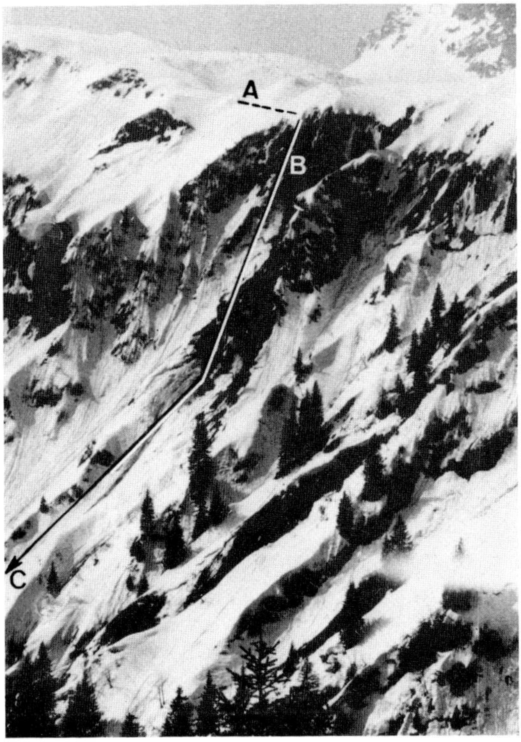

Fig. 2/7. Accident site. A = Ski slope; B = free fall; C = location where found. [Photograph kindly provided by the State police St. Gallen.]

Because a 13-year-old boy (case 13) strayed too far from the slope, he slipped off and tumbled more than 100 m over a rocky precipice, 30 m of it in a free fall (fig. 2/7). He arrived at the hospital in a comatose state. Because of neurological signs, a right craniotomy was performed immediately. Brain contusion with extensive brain swelling developed and called for aggressive surgical procedures. Another patient (case 14, 30-year-old male) slid off the ski slope and fell over a cliff, suffering a severe head injury (fig. 3/22). He was saved by the helicopter rescue service and brought straight to us. He was drowsy and very restless with nasal bleeding and had several bruises on the face. At immediate craniotomy, an extensive epidural hematoma was evacuated (fig. 3/23). Postoperatively, he was intubated and transferred to the intensive recovery ward. The patient made a complete recovery. A third example is that of a 17-year-old female patient (case 15) who fell and slid on the open ski slope and then tumbled more than 10 m. She lost consciousness and was still unconscious 1 h later. After about 2 weeks of conservative treatment, she was discharged from hospital. She has continued to suffer from occasional headaches.

Discussion

At the tops of ski-lifts, there are always boards with maps of the ski slopes, on which the ski slopes are classified from easy to difficult (fig. 2/8). Thus, when visiting a skiing area for the first time, it is very important to choose slopes suitable for the individual skier. It is also important to inform oneself of the geographic layouts, and to keep within slope markers on steep inclines and dangerous curves.

Most skiing areas are divided into 3 degrees of difficulty, the blue, red and black slopes, and those are marked accordingly. Blue means easy, red indicates moderate, and the black ski slope is the most difficult. There are signs indicating dangerous curves on the slope and they are marked by clearly visible boards or nets. When there are snowdrifts or foggy weather, it

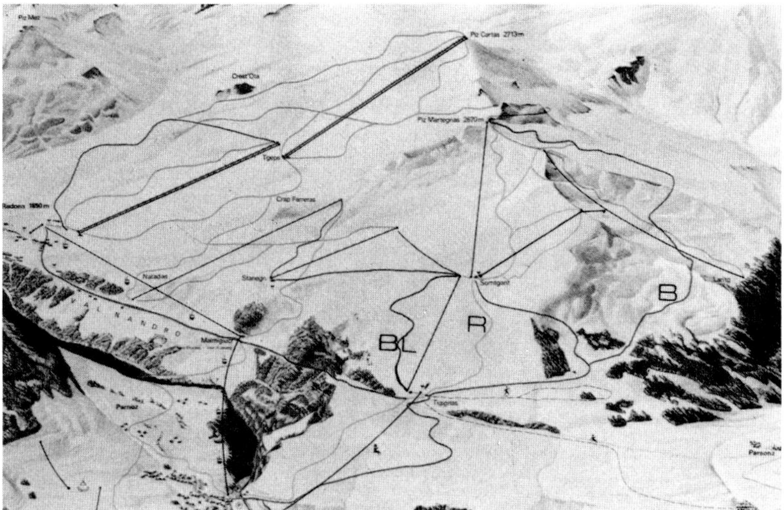

Fig. 2/8. Degrees of difficulty of the ski slopes. B = Blue slope; R = red slope; BL = black slope.

is hard to see these signs and markers, and then serious slipping or sliding accidents often occur.

Skiers who are unfamiliar with the slopes should never ski alone during bad weather, but should go out with experienced skiers who know the slopes well.

Hit by Ski-Lift

These types of head injuries are not uncommon. Direct or indirect blows may cause head injuries, ranging from carelessness leading to being struck by the T-bar (fig. 2/9) through direct blows or being hit by a broken cable of the T-bar to falls from a height onto the head, i.e. an accident from an indirect blow.

Skiers usually make use of the ski-lift for convenience. Carelessness and slow reactions often lead to head injuries caused by direct impact of the T-bars. During the last three skiing seasons (from 1978 to 1981), 14 patients were treated for head injuries resulting from ski-lift accidents (table 2/II).

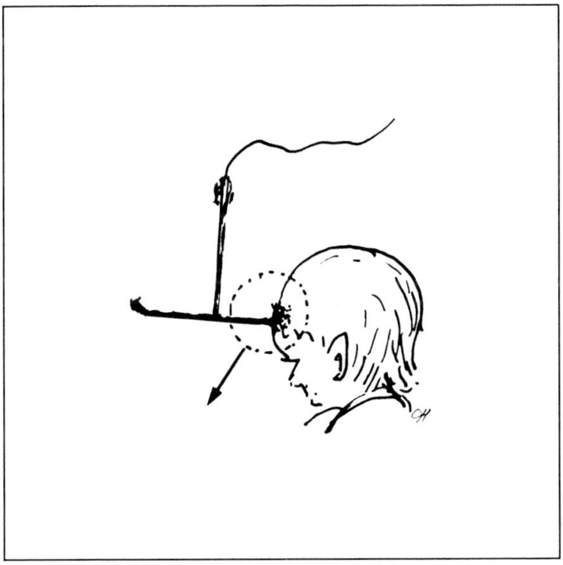

Fig. 2/9. Illustration of head injury caused by ski-lift T-bar.

Table 2/II. Age and sex

Age, years	Men	Women	Total
0–17	3	6	9
18–30	–	–	–
Over 31	–	5	5
Total	3	11	14

Of these, 6 patients were treated surgically for depressed skull fractures. It is noteworthy that these head injuries were mostly suffered by children (65% = 9 cases); women accounted for 80% (11 cases).

A 13-year-old boy (case 16) was hit on his head by a ski-lift T-bar. The patient who was unconscious briefly, was first treated by a local doctor who sutured the open scalp wound and then sent to the hospital. The patient complained of frontal headache and nausea but his reactions were quite normal. He vomited several times during the neurological examination. As time passed, there was gradual deterioration of consciousness and he was finally deeply somnolent. Immediate surgery was performed (fig. 3/26, 27). Postoperative progress was good and he could be discharged without any symptoms 3 weeks later. Case 17 (a 15-year-old boy) suffered a skull fracture from a blow by a ski-lift T-bar (fig. 3/28). He lost consciousness immediately and was brought to us as an emergency. On admission he had regained consciousness. The open depressed fracture was operated at once. A 16-year-old girl (case 18) suffered an indirect head injury during her ride on the ski-lift. She slid downhill for about 300 m and hit her head on the hard ski slope many times (fig. 2/10). She was found in a comatose state. After intubation at the site of the accident, she was transferred to our hospital. Immediate decompressive right craniectomy was carried out. However, the patient died shortly after the decompression operation. This accident caused a fatal indirect head injury.

Discussion

I distinguish between direct and indirect head injuries from ski-lift accidents. Direct injuries are mostly caused by the T-bars striking the head. These accidents may occur because of carelessness, i.e. inappropriate behavior or slow reactions of the patient, or may be caused by another skier.

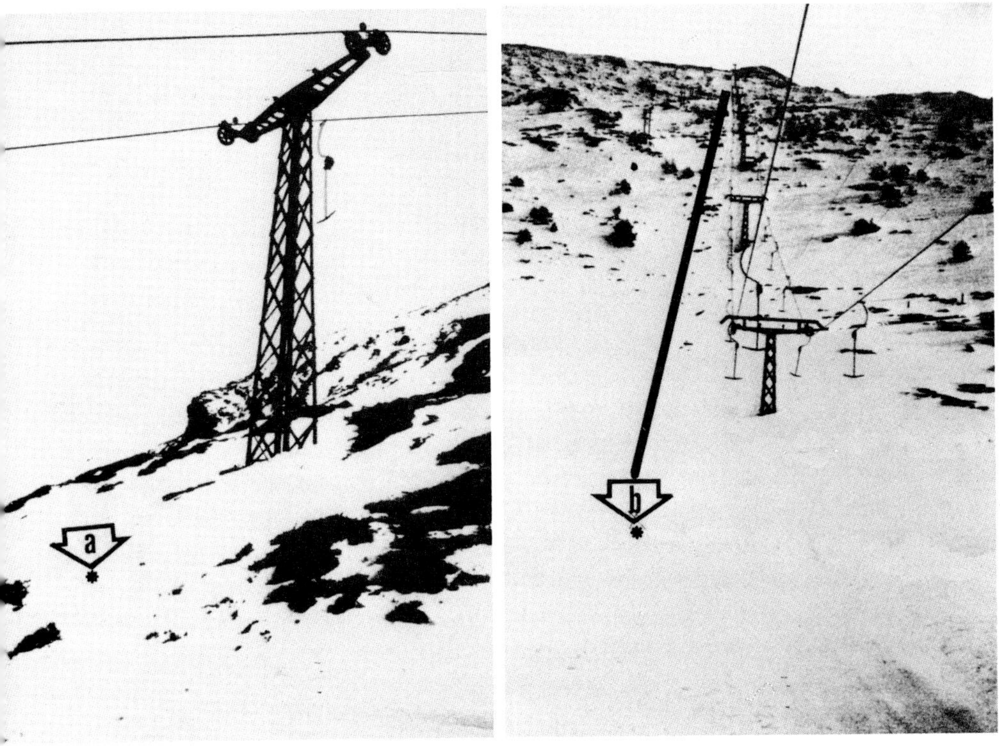

Fig. 2/10. a = Point where fall took place. **b** = Patient located about 300 m from where fall took place.

The smaller the area of impact, the greater the possibility of a depressed skull fracture, which in turn may or may not be accompanied by brain damage. In cases of indirect head injuries from falls when using the ski-lift, trauma to the head occurs secondarily.

Causes of such accidents which may be mentioned are undisciplined use of ski-lift, defective maintenance of ski-lift system (detachment of T-bar cable), inadequate preparation of the ski-lift tracks (worn sections), or icy ski-lift tracks.

Indirect head trauma results in closed brain damage as a rule, and this happened even when the outcome was fatal (case 18). A few cases of post-traumatic epilepsy occurred due to the depressed skull fractures, this unfortunately having a crucial effect on the quality of the patient's subsequent life. Most ski-lift head injuries occurred to children and young skiers.

Collision with Various Obstacles

There is a typical type of head injury resulting from accidents involving various obstacles, namely a depressed skull fracture with or without brain damage due to the impact of energy over a small area [39, 41, 43–45].

This usually occurs off the ski slope after a fall [58]. Excessive speed or speed not adjusted to prevailing conditions often leads to loss of ski control and deviation from the slope, and finally to head injury from colliding with various obstacles.

Wooden railings: A 28-year-old male (case 19) collided with wooden railings. He was skiing at high speed in good weather on powder snow when he lost his balance on a smooth, straight and wide slope shortly before a wooden bridge where there was a fence about 15 m long and 1.5 m high (fig. 2/11). He slid head-first into the wooden bridge railings. He suffered very severe head injuries which caused his death at the site of the accident.

Hidden boulders were the cause of the most serious head injury to a skier that I have ever seen at our hospital.

This 40-year-old man (case 20) skiing on a well-prepared slope in good weather and snow conditions, left the slope and crashed, hitting his head on a boulder (fig. 2/12). The patient became comatose immediately. Despite prompt rescue by helicopter, he died during the flight as a result of his severe head injury.

This fatal head injury was caused in a skiing accident with no-one else involved. Because of the increase in head injuries from skiing, there is a pressing need for simple and direct precautionary measures.

I have already reported this tragic case in a medical journal under the title 'Craniocerebral injuries in skiing and their prevention' [47].

It cannot be repeated too often that preventive medicine is the most up-to-date type of medicine, particularly for head injuries, because substantial progress in the therapy of them is difficult to achieve.

Education in the prevention of injury to the head while skiing (especially the simplest method of direct prevention by wearing a helmet) is thus much more important than the treatment of injuries to the central nervous system, because the former promises better success.

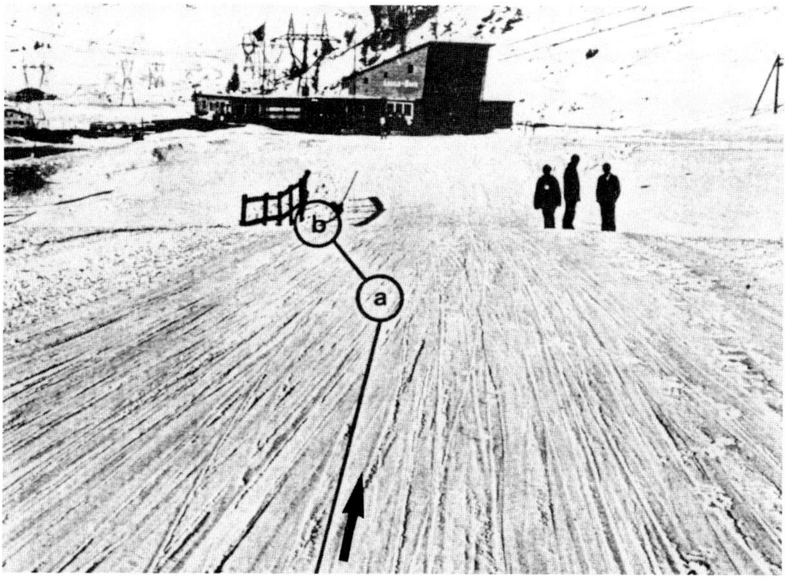

A

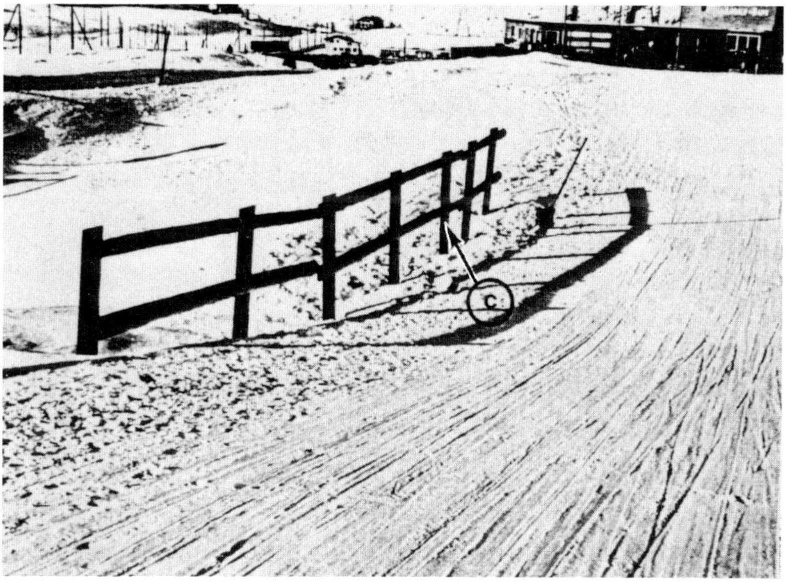

B

Fig. 2/11A, B. Overall view of the site of the accident showing ski path. a = Spot where he slid off; b = point of impact; c = close-up spot where crash occurred. [Photographs kindly provided by the State police of Graubünden.]

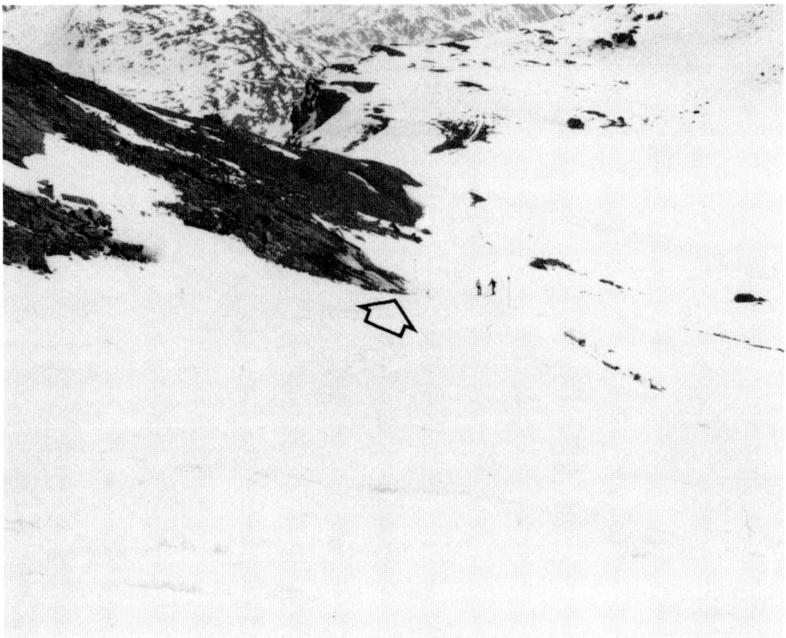

Fig. 2/12. Accident site. [Photograph provided by the State police of Graubünden.]

Collision accidents with rocks may involve either snow-covered or bare rocks. Though collision with a bare rock obviously involves a skiing error, the case of cliffs or rocks which are hidden by fresh snow or beneath poorly prepared slopes is especially dangerous. These nonvisible rocks stop the skier abruptly, frequently resulting in a fall where the head directly hits a sharp rock (fig. 2/13).

For example, a 21-year-old man (case 21) was skiing with four friends on fresh snow, fell over a snow-hidden rock, and suffered an open head injury. He did not lose consciousness and was admitted to the hospital with complaints of headache and nausea. Though his only physical sign was a small cut, a skull X-ray (fig. 3/36) showed a depressed fracture requiring immediate surgery.

In another case, a 12-year-old boy (case 22) fell on the slope and went into a slide that was violently stopped when his head hit a rock. He lost consciousness immediately, was transported by helicopter to our hospital where he underwent emergency surgery (fig. 3/37, 38). After 4 weeks of

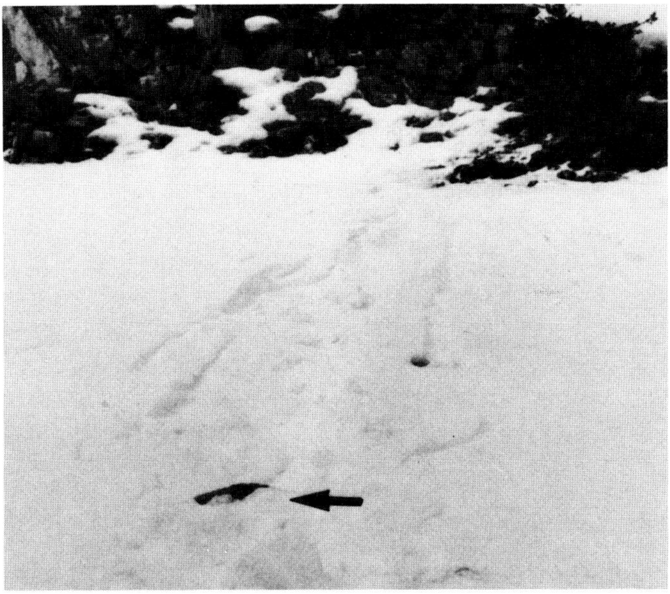

Fig. 2/13. Rock hidden by fresh snow.

hospitalization, the patient was discharged in generally good condition, though a second surgical operation was performed a few months later for cosmetic reasons.

A third example illustrates the increased risk of head injuries paradoxically created by the superb functioning of safety bindings. This 20-year-old man (case 23) fell while skiing on fresh snow. Both skis were released automatically, and the man was thrown headfirst against a rock. Surgical treatment was successful, and the man was discharged without complications following 3 weeks of hospitalization under conservative treatment. However, as is often the case with severe head injuries, later complications arose and the patient was again admitted for surgical treatment by CSF fistula (fig. 3/40).

Ski-lift mast: Head injury caused by collision with the ski-lift mast is rare. It usually causes forehead injuries (fig. 2/14). One such case is that of a 36-year-old man (case 24) who fell one afternoon crashing his head against a

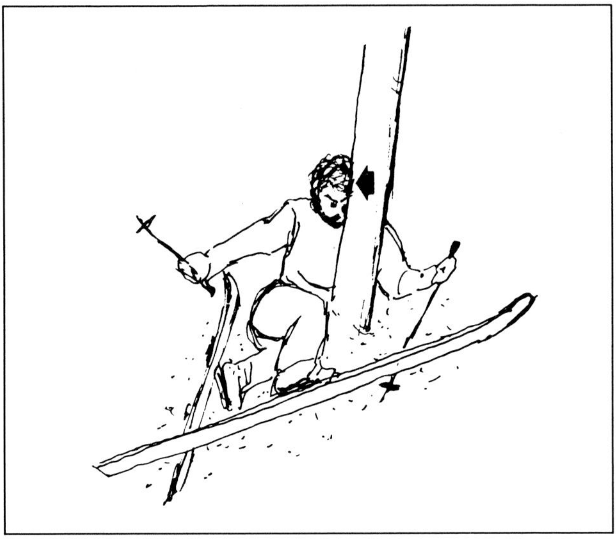

Fig. 2/14. Collision with ski-lift mast causing serious head injury.

ski-lift mast. He lost consciousness immediately. First aid was given at the local hospital, and he was then transferred to us for emergency surgery, which was carried out immediately. He recovered completely within 3 weeks of the injury (fig. 2/14).

Collisions with stones: Insufficient snow on the open ski slope often causes collisions with stones. The head crashes against stones after falling. For example, a 15-year-old male (case 25) lost control while skiing at speed and fell on the slope and rolled over many times, hitting his head on the ground and then on stone. On his way to the hospital he vomited several times. He was drowsy. A large scalp wound was present and a depressed fracture was felt underneath it. We could reposition the fracture perfectly. There were no postoperative complications. Another case (case 26) was of a 10-year-old boy who was skiing carelessly and fast when he lost control and fell on the open slope. His head crashed against the slope which did not have much snow. The boy could not remember the cause of the accident. He vomited many times on the way to hospital. A closed depressed fracture (fig. 3/44) was repaired 5 days later by surgical repositioning. There were no postoperative complications.

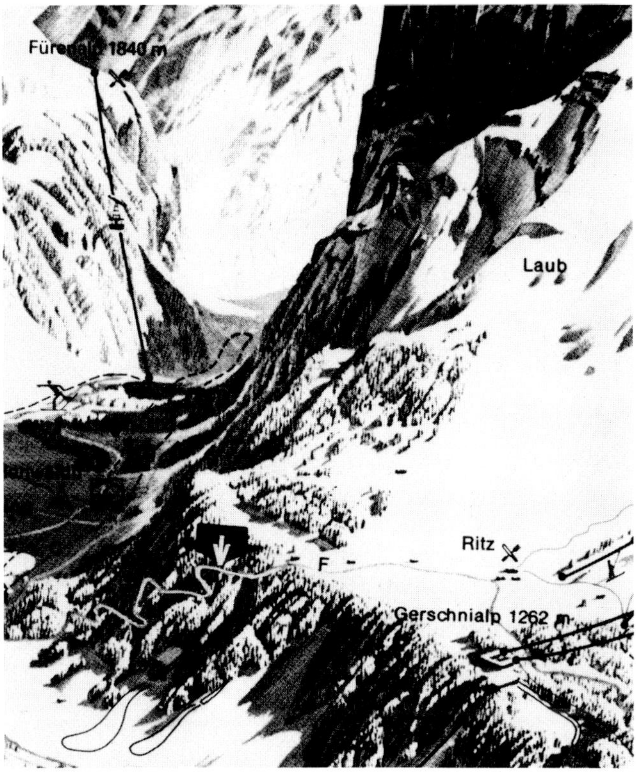

Fig. 2/15. Narrow forest path.

Concrete base of a pole: A 12-year-old boy (case 27) fell on the open ski slope and then slid off, hitting his head against the concrete base of a pole. He was somnolent for a few hours after the accident. He had an open depressed fracture (fig. 3/45) which was treated by immediate surgery. Postoperative course was good and the patient was discharged symptom-free 12 days later. A bone defect was repaired 3 months later.

Collision with trees: Narrow forest paths on the way to villages (fig. 2/15), slope-connecting paths, and slopes alongside woods give rise to the danger of collision with trees, especially when there is traffic congestion during late afternoon before the ski-lift is closed, with many skiers on the way home. These accidents are common and mostly cause frontal head injuries (fig. 2/16).

2/16

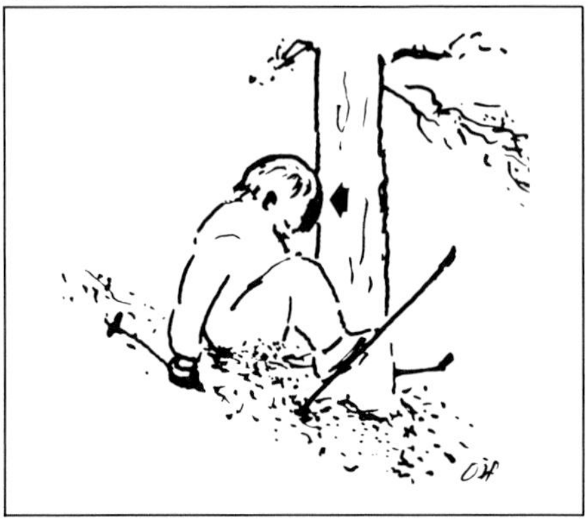

2/17

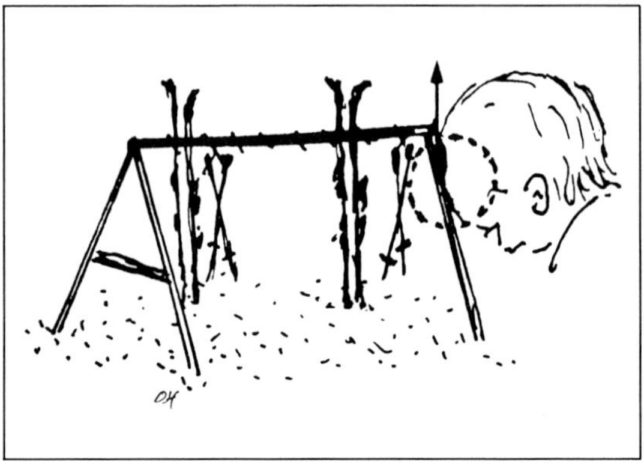

Fig. 2/16. Collision with a tree.
Fig. 2/17. Collision with ski rack.

An 11-year-old girl (case 28) crashed head-on into a tree on a forest path. She was unconscious and was first taken to the district hospital. She was later transferred to us for surgery (fig. 3/46). We were able to reposition the depressed fracture which had occurred and the patient made a complete recovery.

Collision with a ski rack is rare. A 17-year-old patient (case 29), according to eye witnesses, crashed his head into a ski rack (fig. 2/17). After the accident, he was unconscious and vomited many times. He was admitted to the local hospital as an emergency case. Spontaneous restlessness appeared and progressed until he lapsed in deep unconsciousness. Due to the possibility of intracranial hemorrhage, he was transferred to us, where he was subsequently operated. Postoperative progress was slow but satisfactory. 6 days later he was awake and responsive. Due to left hemiparesis he had to undergo intense physiotherapy. He was later transferred to a hospital nearer his home for continuation of the physiotherapy.

Hitting a wall: The aerial cable station is usually located in the middle of the skiing area. From the top cable station or beginning of the ski-lift, the route home leads through forest (fig. 2/15), over bridges, and past some small alpine huts (fig. 2/18). By losing control at high speed on the narrow path, skiers occasionally fall and crash into a hard wall (wood or concrete) and suffer craniocerebral injuries (fig. 2/19). Skiing along a narrow path to

2/18 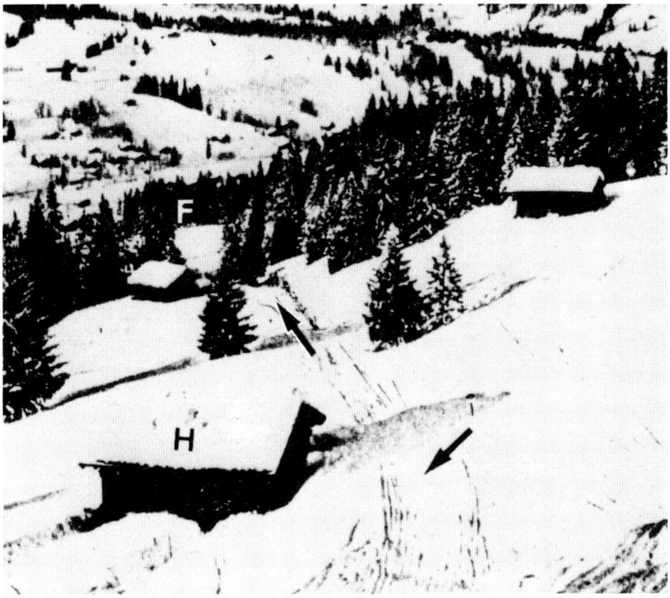

2/19 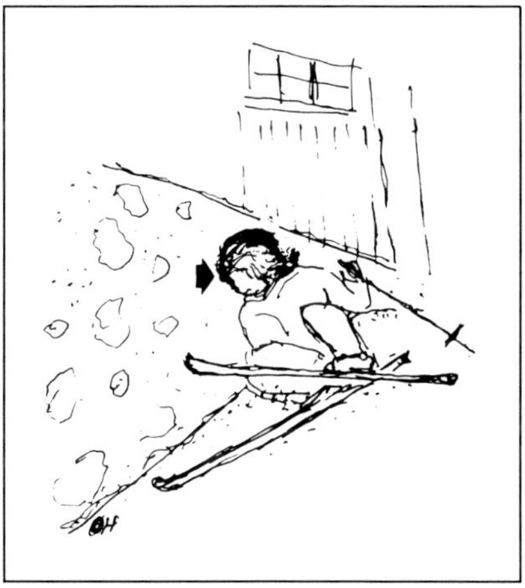

Fig. 2/18. The way home leads through forest and past huts (H).
Fig. 2/19. Head hitting against wall.

another ski slope, a 53-year-old male (case 30) crashed straight into the concrete wall of a mountain hut hitting his head violently. He lost consciousness immediately. He was able to answer questions coherently 3 days later and after 3 weeks he was discharged from the hospital in good general condition.

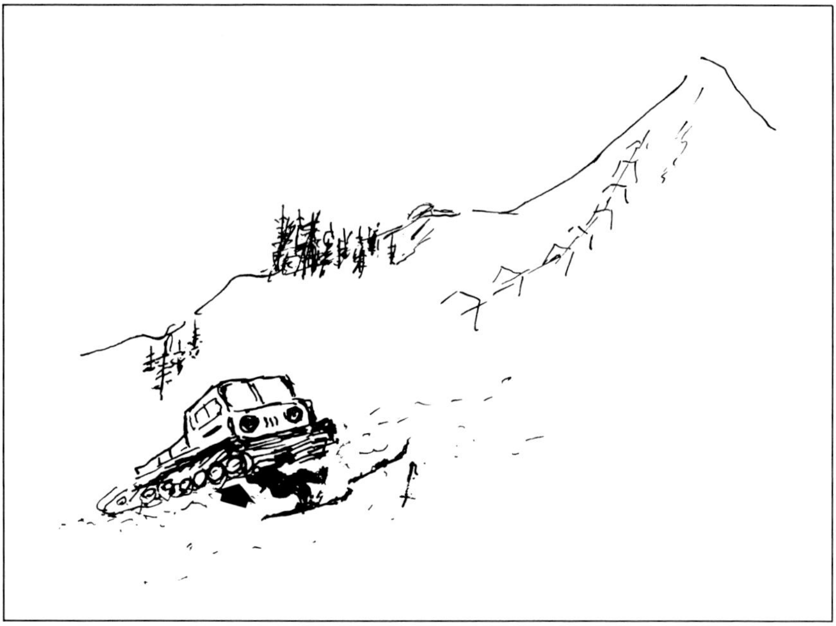

Fig. 2/20. Illustration of accident situation.

Collision with a snowplough: A 16-year-old girl fell on the ski slope and collided with a snowplough (case 31). She strangulated her head completely (fig. 2/20). She was later found, unconscious and with respiratory arrest. She was given artificial respiration and was transferred to our hospital by helicopter. She regained consciousness 24 h later after being given antiedematous medication and artificial respiration. 4 days later, she was transferred to a hospital in Germany at her family's request.

Unknown Causes

I shall give examples of these unknown causes with 3 cases. The first, a 30-year-old male (case 32), came from Germany. He was found unconscious beside the ski slope, and was then transported to us by helicopter. During immediate surgery (fig. 3/52, 53), we found dural laceration with brain damage. The second was a 20-year-old male (case 33) who was found in an unconscious state one morning near the slope. He was rushed to the hospital by helicopter where he was given first aid. After examination, an immediate craniectomy (fig. 3/55, 56) was performed. Despite the immediate surgical treatment, the patient died a few days later. The third was a 14-year-old male (case 34) who fell while skiing. He was sent to us by helicopter. There was slow and progressive deterioration from consciousness to coma. Craniectomy was performed. This seemed to be successful but 4 days later he started showing signs of deterioration again, he was comatose for more than 2 weeks. Despite intensive care, his condition worsened progressively and he died 2 months later.

It is not uncommon for the causes of skiing accidents to be unknown. If the skier is alone and loses consciousness due to head injury, the cause of the accident is unknown. There are no spectators. Did the accident involve only the injured skier or not? It is ideal if at least 3 skiers go out together: they can enjoy companionship and assist each other. Furthermore, if an accident happens, they know the cause of it and they can help with first aid.

Discussion

I have dealt with the various causes of skiing accidents involving the head, such as head-to-head collisions, impact by items of ski equipment with small surface areas, ski-lift T-bar accidents, various obstacles, etc., resulting mostly in depressed skull fractures (penetrating injuries), accompanied by brain damage.

The depressed fractures usually required neurosurgical treatment and my clinical experience has shown that 84% (children 92%) of surgical cases are caused by skiing accidents. What must be the nature and shape of the impinging object and the type of collision to cause depressed fractures of the skull, and how strong must the force be? Why is there depression of the fractured pieces? I have studied these questions clinically and experimentally, as may be seen in the article, the 'Experimental study of depressed fractures and structures' [43, 45, 49].

Parallel with this I concentrated my studies on the simplest measure to prevent head injuries using the ideal functional protection, that is the *helmet*. The prevention of penetrating injuries to the skull associated with brain damage, which are typical of recent skiing accidents and require operative procedures, is actually easy and simple: by wearing a curved, hard, glazed, light, plastic ski-helmet! I am a great fan of skiing, because to me it is the most pleasant and healthy recreation during the long winter [2].

3 Case Reports and Statistical Data

Free Fall

Case 1

Male, 42 years old (minor accident). The patient suffered a minor fall on an open slope about 4 weeks prior to coming to our hospital. He visited a local hospital on the day of the accident, where slight brain contusion was found. Since then he had complained of occasional minor headaches. 2 days before admission, the patient had sudden, increasingly severe, bitemporal headaches with dizziness and nausea. The patient was first admitted to the district hospital. Here they found a steady deterioration in consciousness (drowsiness) without any neurological deficits, for which reason the patient was transferred to us for further examination. On admission, the patient was deeply unconscious with respiratory disturbances. Papilledema and bilateral Babinski reflex were found. The echoencephalogram revealed slight displacement of the midline from left to right. A left carotid angiogram (fig. 3/1) showed inward displacement of the surface vessels from the skull by the subdural hematomas, with no displacement of the anterior cerebral artery. The pattern is that of a typical chronic bilateral subdural hematoma. Surgery revealed extensive chronic bilateral hemorrhage. Postoperatively, his clinical condition was satisfactory, and he was discharged 3 weeks later without any symptoms.

Case 2

Female, 54 years old. A woman, while skiing on a soft slope, had suffered a minor fall with mild concussion. No medical care was sought. As time went on, the patient suffered from recurrent mild headaches at irregular intervals. Shortly before hospitalization the woman experienced difficulty in writing and she found that she dropped things more often. On admission, 4 weeks after the accident, she had slight speech disturbances

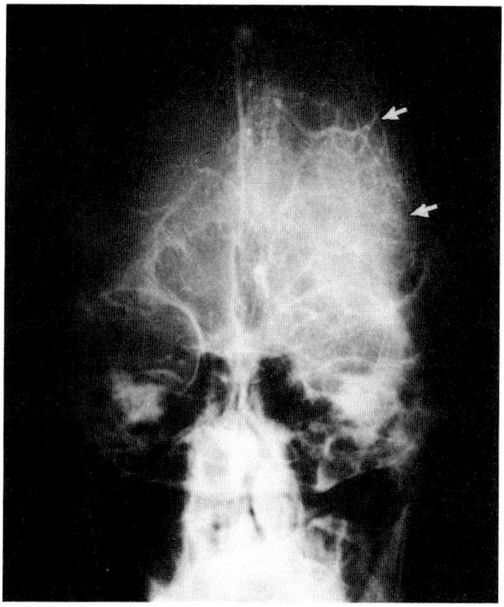

Fig. 3/1. Avascular space due to chronic bilateral subdural hematoma.

and arithmetic difficulties. No obvious neurological signs. Lumbar puncture resulted in clear CSF, and the pressure, the cell count and the protein value were normal. An electroencephalogram showed a low-arched curve, which showed a left cerebral hemisphere and very irregularly a slight accumulation of delta waves.

Because of the pathological EEG finding, a further examination by computed tomography of the brain was performed. Surprisingly, the CT image revealed a large chronic subdural hemorrhage in the left hemisphere (fig. 3/2). The hematoma could be removed (without any problems) via two burr holes. The woman was discharged 4 weeks after the operation. 3 months later, at an outpatient check-up she had no more headaches and was completely free of any discomfort.

Case 3

Male, 26 years old. The patient fell on an open hard snow slope and immediately became unconscious. A convulsive seizure occurred, and then he became deeply comatose, which led to emergency transfer to our neuro-

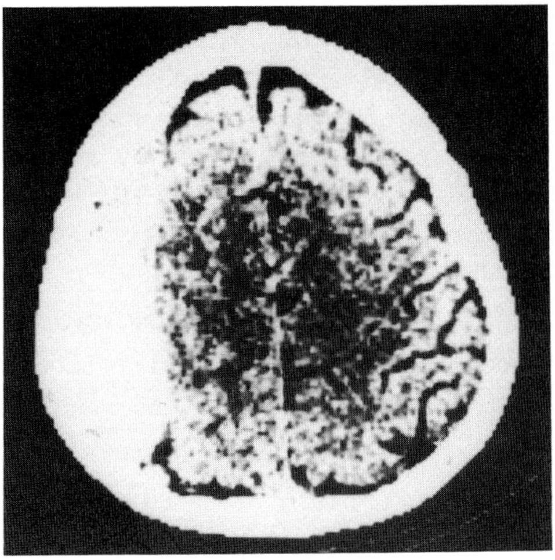

Fig. 3/2. Large chronic subdural hematoma on the left.

surgical department. A superficial bruise on the right forehead and face, and leakage of CSF from the right ear were found. Except for bilateral Babinski reflexes there were no other neuropathological findings. The skull X-ray revealed a linear fracture in the right temporobasal region (fig. 3/3). After 3 weeks of conservative medical care, his condition was good. On discharge from hospital, he had a disturbance of hearing on the right.

Case 4

Male, 24 years old. The patient fell on a hard, icy ski slope and suffered a brain contusion with immediate unconsciousness. On admission, a fixed, dilated right pupil with progressive loss of consciousness was found. The skull X-ray showed a right linear fracture in the parietotemporal area extending to the basal region (fig. 3/4). An immediate right carotid angiogram revealed a large avascular space in the parietotemporal region due to an epidural hematoma (fig. 3/5A, B). The patient underwent immediate surgery. During the operation a large epidural hematoma was found, and

---

Fig. 3/3. Right temporobasal fracture with otorrhea.

Fig. 3/4. Large skull fracture in the right parietal extending to the basal region.

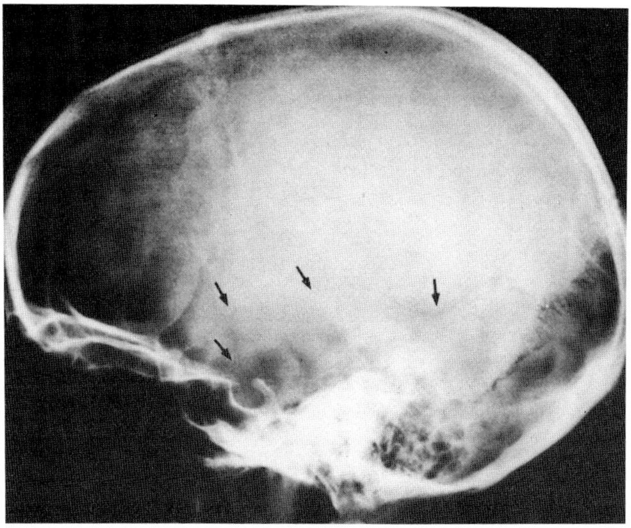

3/3

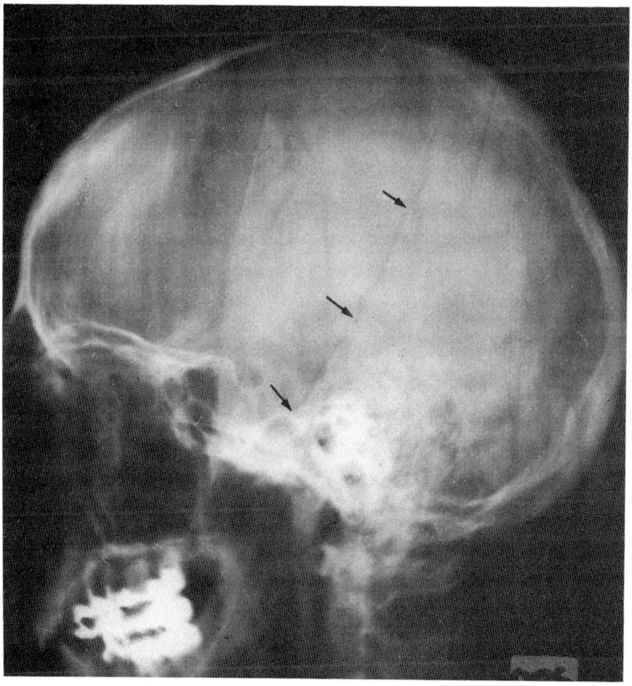

3/4

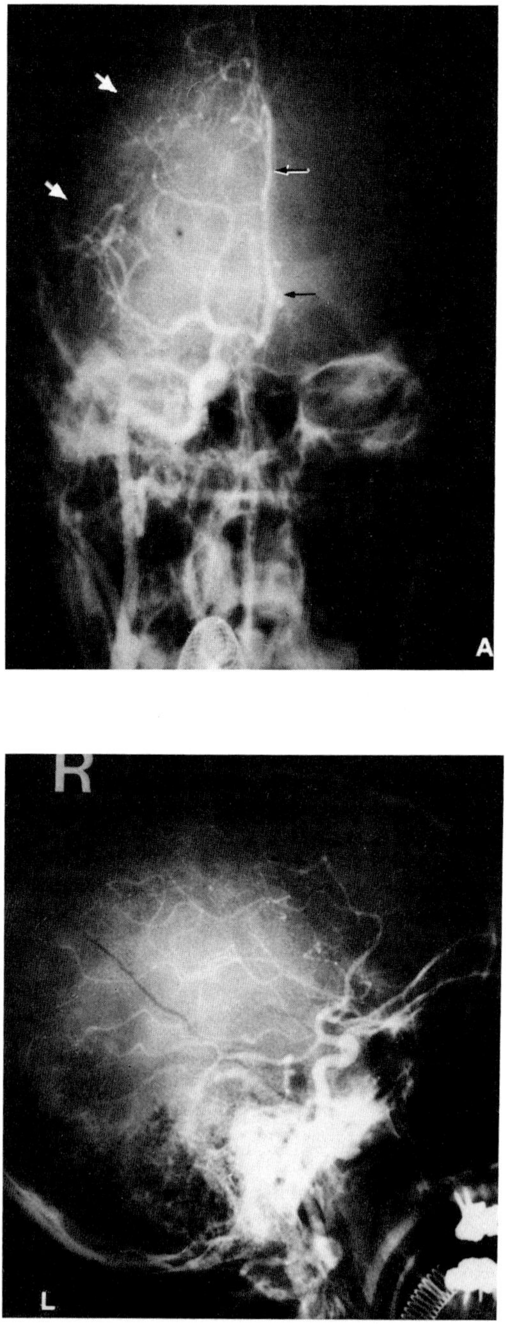

A

B

Fig. 3/5. A AP view; **B** lateral view. Avascular space in right parietal region with displacement of cerebral vessels due to epidural hemorrhage (**A**) and extensive linear fracture (**B**).

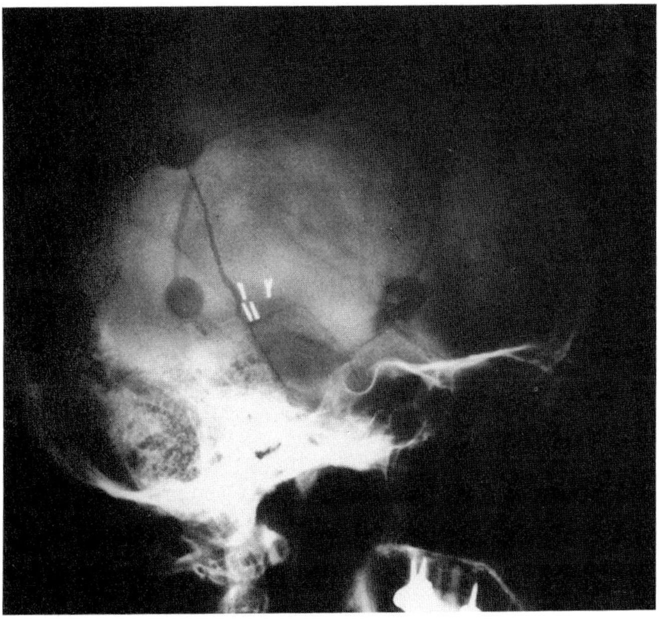

Fig. 3/6. Postoperative finding.

was evacuated by craniotomy (fig. 3/6). The condition of the patient after the operation improved so much that he could be discharged without any symptoms about 4 weeks later. Later, he suffered a convulsive seizure (grand mal), so that continuous anticonvulsive medication is necessary.

Case 5

Male, 17 years old. The patient fell on an open slope due to losing his balance. He immediately became unconscious and was transferred to us as an emergency. On admission he was somnolent with both Babinski signs. There were no other neurological deficits, in particular no pathological findings on the pupils. The left side of the neck showed an extensive bruise, as did the right side of the forehead. X-rays of skull and cervical spine revealed no fractures. Brain contusion was diagnosed and the patient was treated conservatively. The patient was discharged with a postcontusion syndrome about 3 weeks later. The patient suffered from occasional headaches which were monitored as an outpatient.

3 years later the patient consulted me now suffering from continuous dull headaches and deterioration in memory. CT scanning surprisingly

showed a serious communicating hydrocephalus aresorptiva (fig. 3/7). Surgical treatment was then performed to construct a ventriculo-abdominal shunt. The patient no longer complains of headaches and his memory functions better now. The slight disturbances in psycho-organic functions have also disappeared completely.

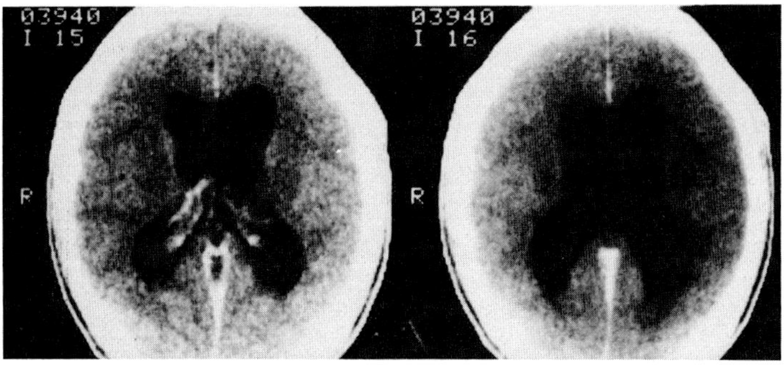

Fig. 3/7. CT scan showing a serious internal hydrocephalus malresorptiva.

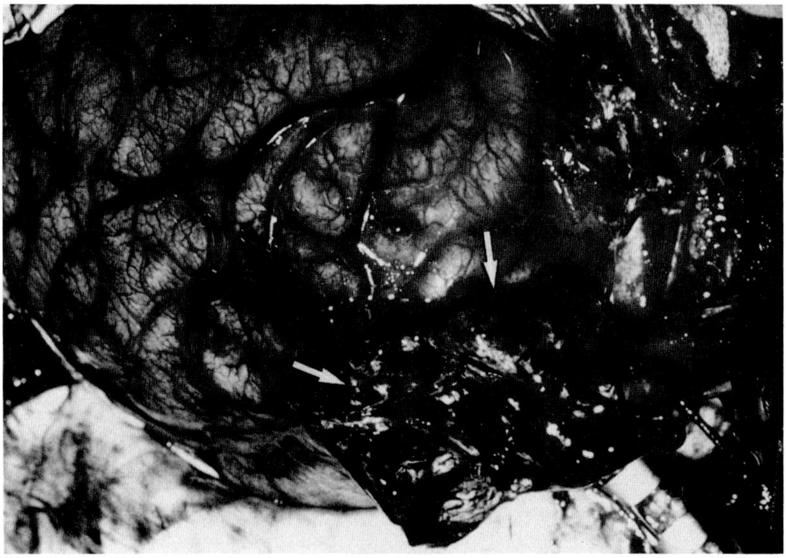

Fig. 3/8. Extended brain damage with hemorrhage in the right parietotemporal area and extensive brain edema (finding at operation).

Case 6

Male, 17 years old. The patient injured himself in an accident jumping at high speed while skiing. Immediately after the accident, consciousness became impaired and he rapidly became more somnolent. On emergency admission to hospital the patient was deeply comatose and the pupils remained moderately dilated and did not respond to light stimuli. Neurological examination showed a midbrain syndrome. Respiration was impaired, so the patient was intubated at once. The echoencephalogram revealed a slight displacement of the midline from the right to the left. Based on the pathological echoencephalogram, a right craniectomy was performed immediately. It showed an extended brain contusion with noxious brain edema (fig. 3/8). Despite aggressive surgical treatment, the patient died 2 days later of central respiratory and cardiac arrest following severe brain damage.

Collision with Another Skier

Case 7

18-year-old male (a) collided with 43-year-old male (b). Head to head collision of the 2 patients on an open slope, and both immediately became unconscious (fig. 3/9). Patient a received an extended, closed depressed

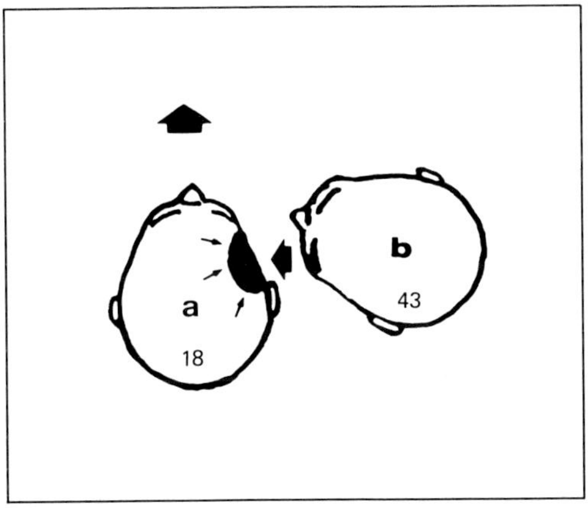

Fig. 3/9. Severely injured (a) suffered extensive right temporal depressed fracture.

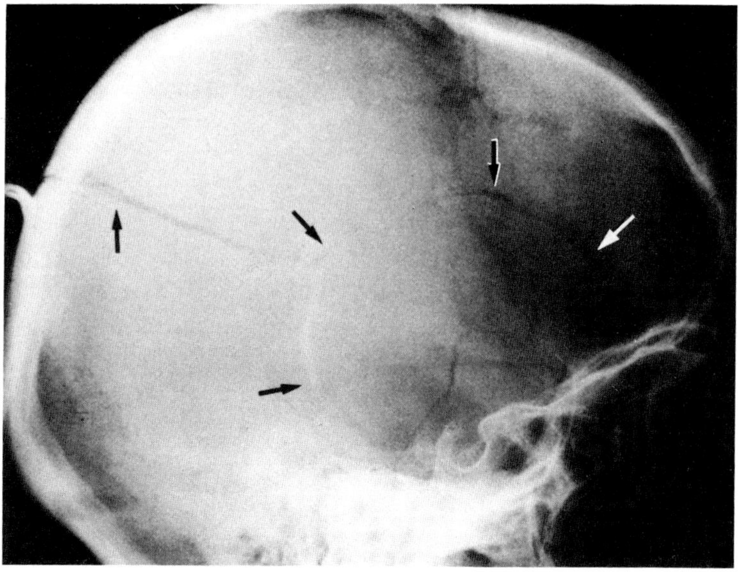

3/10

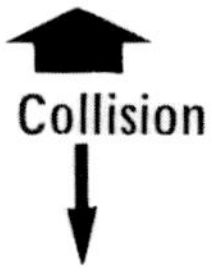

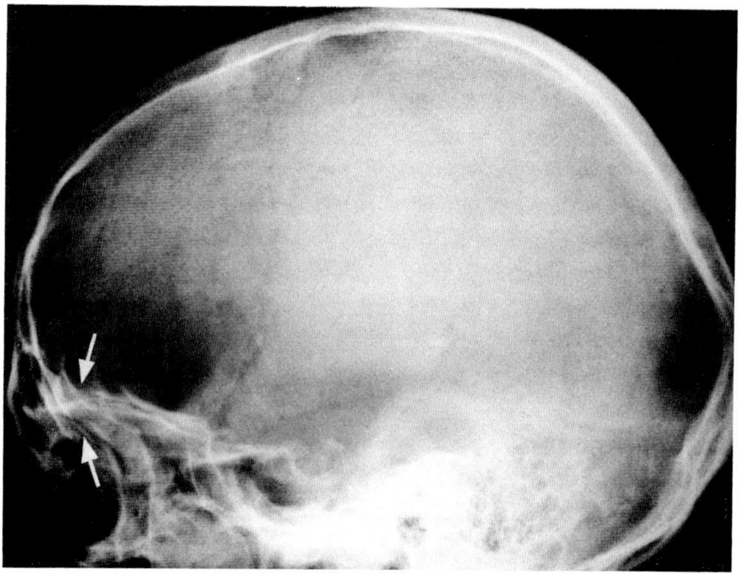

3/11

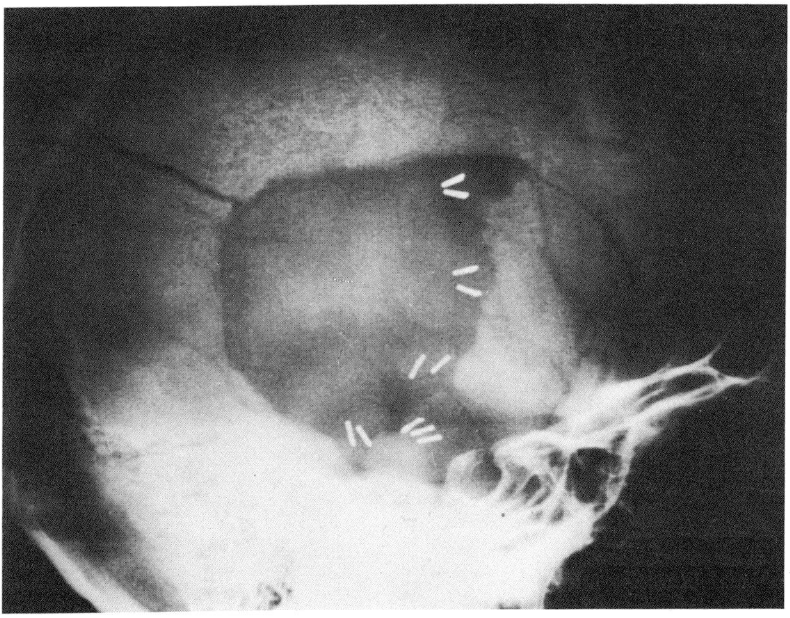

Fig. 3/12. Postoperative skull defect.

parietal fracture on the right, as well as severe brain contusions. He was brought to us by helicopter as an emergency. On admission, the patient had developed left hemiparesis accompanied by stupor and with the right pupil slightly dilated and fixed. There was rapid deterioration of consciousness with a left Babinski sign. Skull X-ray showed an extended star-shaped depressed fracture in the right temporal area and a right parietal linear fracture (fig. 3/10). From the neurological findings, an epidural hematoma was suspected. Emergency right craniectomy showed an extended epidural hematoma in the area of the depressed fracture. I carefully debrided the depressed bone fragments (fig. 3/12) and evacuated an epidural blood clot about 3 cm thick. The dural bleeding point (lacerated meningeal artery) was well controlled with clips. The subdural space showed slight

---

Fig. 3/10. Extensive star-shaped right temporal depressed fracture and linear parietal fracture (severely injured).

Fig. 3/11. Left frontobasal fracture (slightly injured).

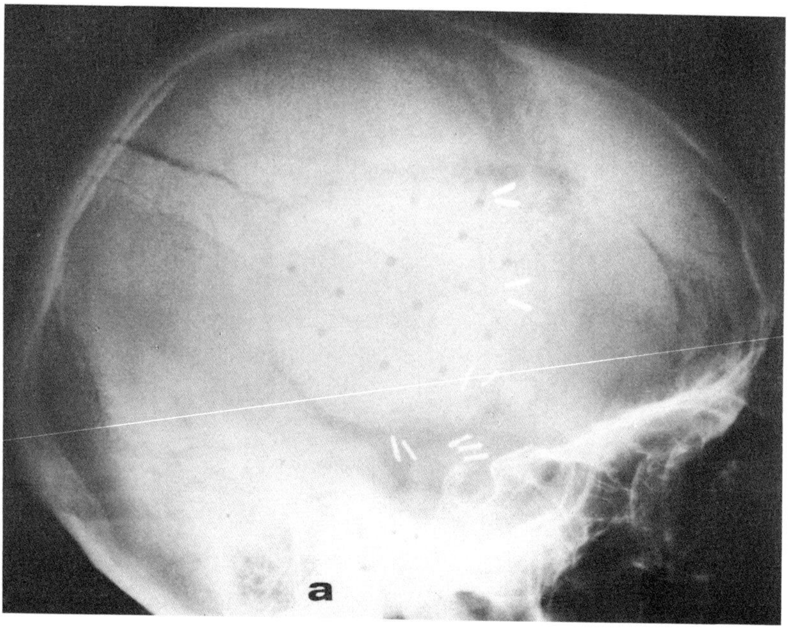

Fig. 3/13. Palacos cranioplasty of the skull defect.

brain contusion. The postoperative course was good, and 3 weeks later he was discharged with posttraumatic complaints, such as occasional headache and dizziness. Neurologically, there was still a slight central facial paresis on the left as well as distinct left hemiparesis. 2 months later, the patient was admitted again for repair of the larger bone defect after surgical treatment of the depressed skull fracture with epidural hematoma. The bone defect was repaired by Palacos cranioplasty (fig. 3/13).

Patient b suffered a frontobasal skull fracture with a slight brain contusion (fig. 3/11). He was treated conservatively for 2 weeks and subsequently sent home free of symptoms.

Case 8

11-year-old female collided with 14-year-old male. In a fall on the ski slope the girl suffered a fracture of the left lower leg. She was unable to get up and remained lying on the ski slope. Shortly afterwards, another skier (14-year-old boy) collided with the girl lying on the ground in such a careless way that he hit the girl's head at full speed. The tip of his ski hit the girl's

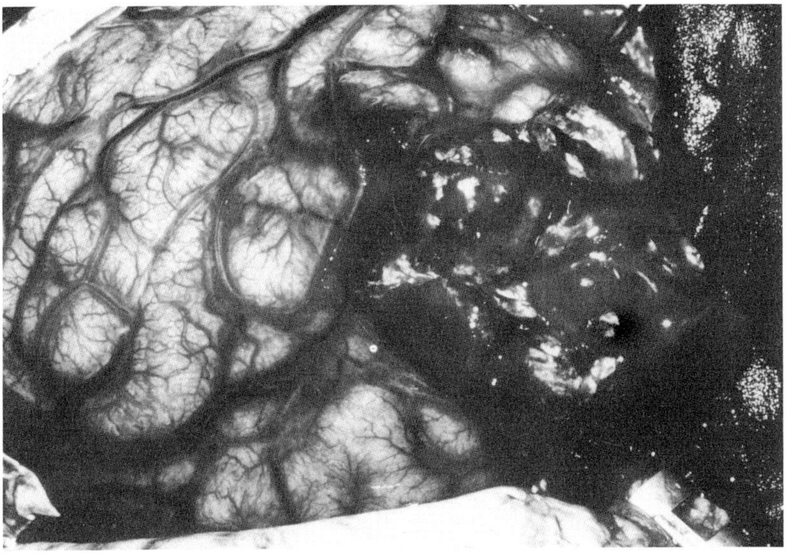

Fig. 3/14. Extensive right occipital brain contusion.

head, causing an open comminuted compound depressed fracture in the right occipital region with severe brain contusion (fig. 3/14). Despite aggressive surgical treatment, i.e. extensive decompressive craniectomy removing much of the damaged brain tissues and open ventricular CSF drainage, and large doses of antiedematous drugs and hyperventilation attempts, the girl died 2 days later due to cardiac and circulatory arrest as a result of the severe brain injury (fig. 3/15A–C).

Case 9

Male, 46 years old. The patient was skiing carefully and slowly on an open slope. A 15-year-old boy ran into him at high speed causing severe head injuries from the collision (fig. 3/16). Both patients were admitted together as emergencies. The 15-year-old boy (fig. 3/16, b) suffered a slight brain contusion and after 9 days of conservative treatment was discharged without any symptoms. The other patient (fig. 3/16, a), severely injured, received a severe open head injury: neurological examination showed 3rd right cranial nerve injury and bilateral Babinski signs. He was somnolent

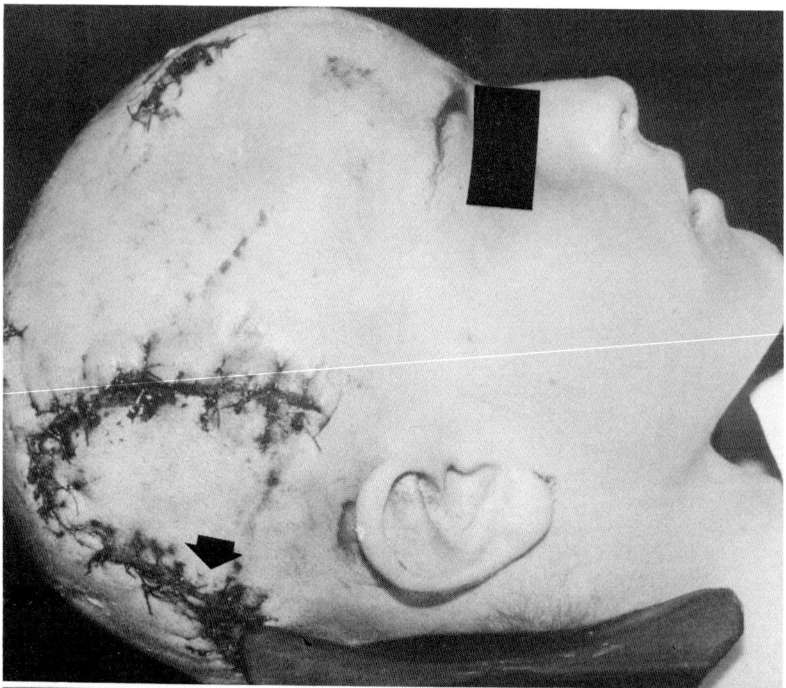

3/15A

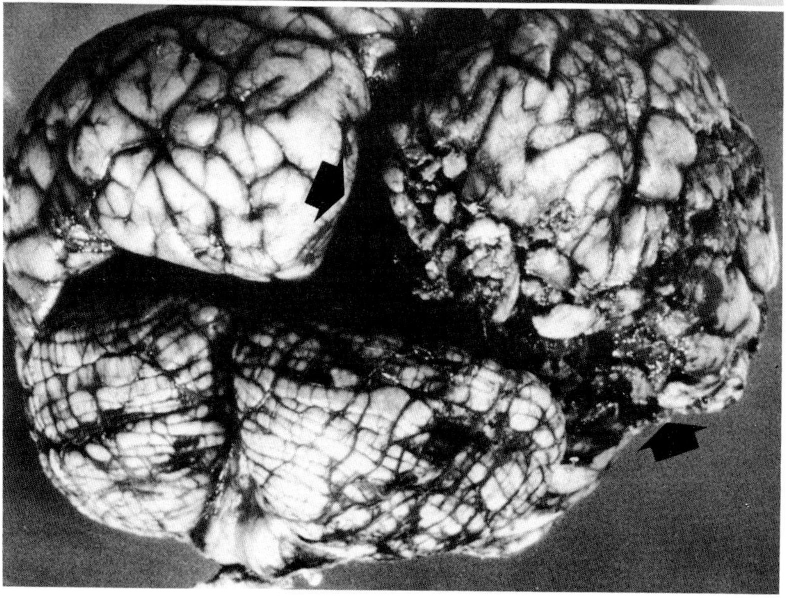

3/15B

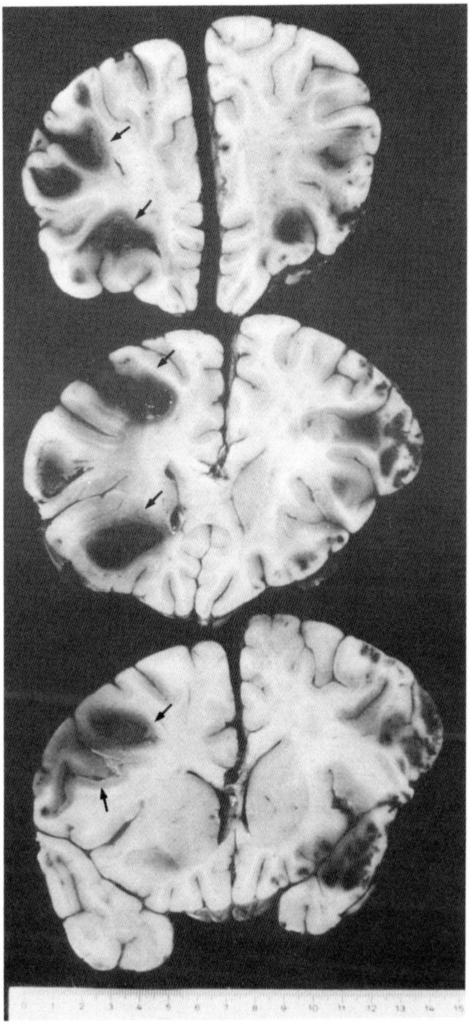

3/15C

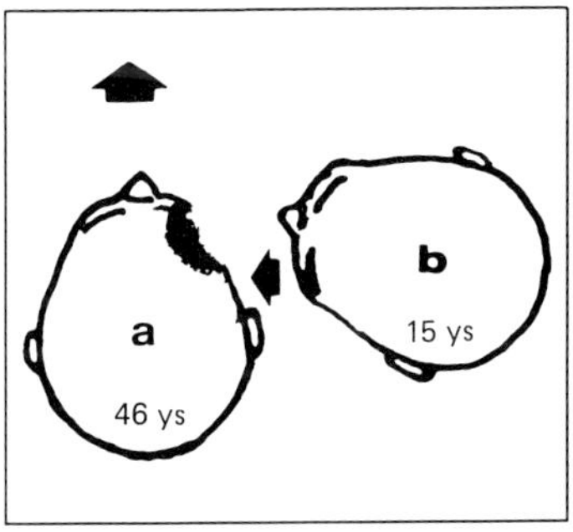

3/16

Fig. 3/15. A Autopsy showed an extensive right occipital brain contusion as well as extensive brain damage on the opposite side. **B** Extensive contusion of the right occipital lobe. **C** Extensive brain contusion on the opposite side (contre-coup).

Fig. 3/16. Illustration of accident: (a) suffered right frontal open depressed skull fracture.

A B

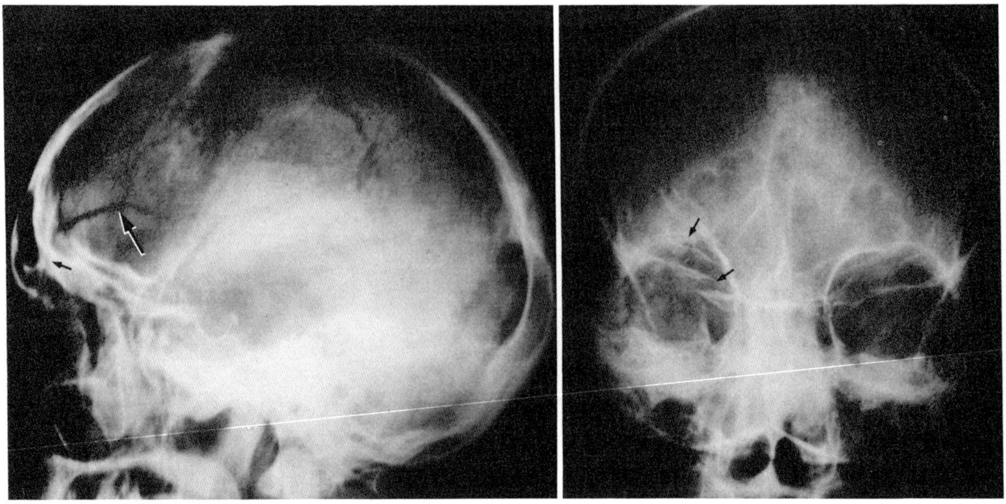

Fig. 3/17A, B. Right frontobasal depressed fracture, with orbital fracture.

A B

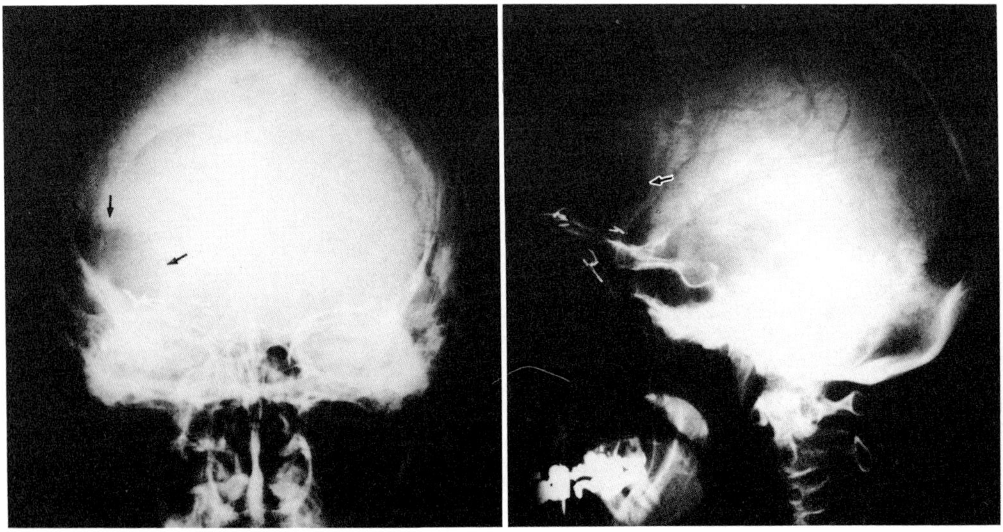

Fig. 3/18A, B. Defect of skull bone after craniectomy (**A**) and wire fixation of the orbital fracture (**B**).

and bleeding from the nose. A scalp wound on the right frontal area was seen. Skull X-ray showed a depressed right frontobasal fracture with orbital fracture (fig. 3/17A, B). Surgery was immediately performed. The depressed fragments were debrided and the unstable fracture of the right orbital bone underwent wire fixation (fig. 3/18A, B).

Injury Caused by Ski Equipment

Case 10

Male, 24 years old. The patient fell on an open slope, and the tip of his ski struck his head, he suffered brief amnesia. An open left parietal depressed skull fracture was found (fig. 3/19A, B). Right Babinski sign. No other neurological signs were checked. The open depressed fracture required immediate surgery to remove depressed bone fragments and repair minor tears in the dura mater. After 12 postoperative days he could be sent home to Germany where a cranioplasty will be done at a later date.

Case 11

Male, 37 years old. The patient fell while skiing and the handle of the ski stick happened to hit his right eye. The patient underwent a brief period of restless unconsciousness, and was transferred to us as an emergency. The right eyelid was found to be greatly swollen with laceration of the eyeball. The

A B

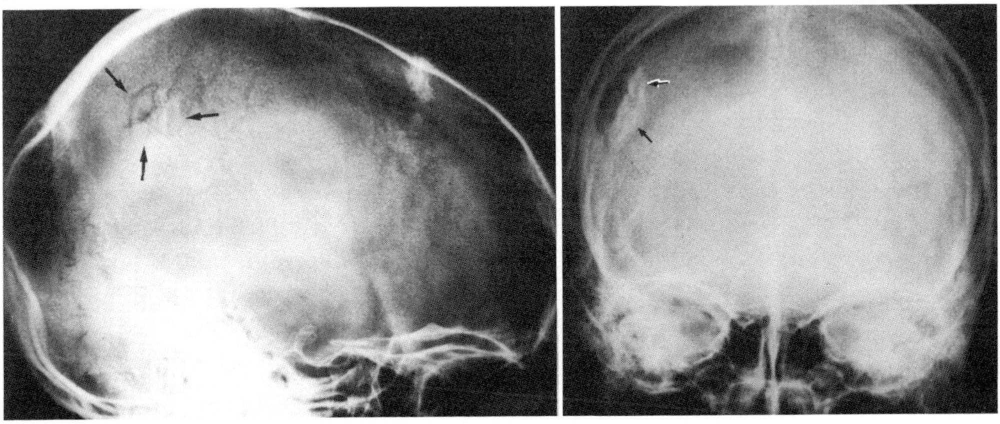

Fig. 3/19A, B. Open depressed fracture caused by tip of own ski. **A** Lateral view; **B** AP view.

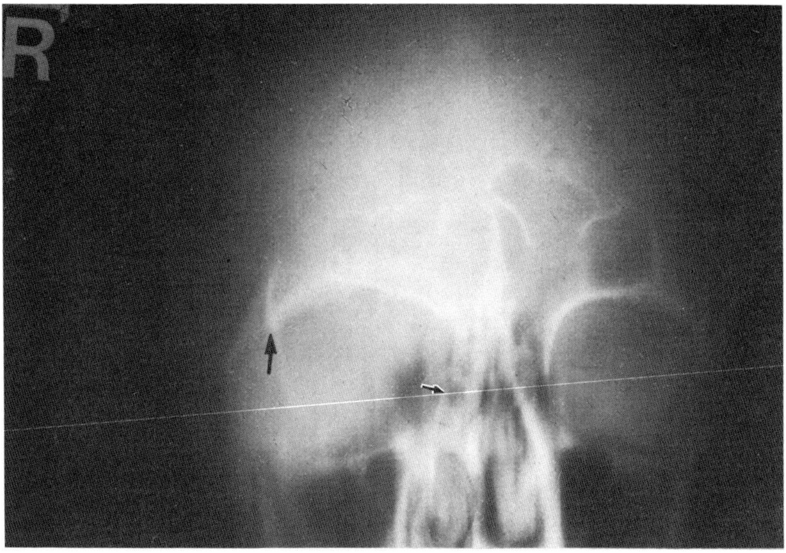

Fig. 3/20. Right displaced supraorbital ridge fracture and fracture of the nasal ethmoid complex.

X-rays revealed a supraorbital ridge fracture with downward displacement (fig. 3/20). Enucleation of the right eye was performed first, and later an open reduction of the displaced fracture of the supraorbital ridge with wire fixation was performed. In the middle, a nasal ethmoid sinus fracture with dural rupture was found, and this was repaired to prevent a CSF fistula.

Case 12

Male, 15 years old. The patient fell on the open slope and the sharp end of the ski stick hit his forehead. He lost consciousness briefly. Immediate first aid was given by rescuers who found an open wound above the right eye. Skull X-ray showed a complete open depressed skull fracture under the laceration (fig. 3/21A, B). A CT scan showed a displaced fracture fragment in the brain (fig. 3/21C) and the fracture communicated with the right frontal sinus (fig. 3/21D). Immediate surgical treatment was performed. At

---

Fig. 3/21A–D. Open depressed fracture above the right eye. **A** Lateral view. **B** AP view. CT scan; complete displaced fracture fragment in the brain (**C**) and fracture communicating with the frontal sinus (**D**).

3/21A

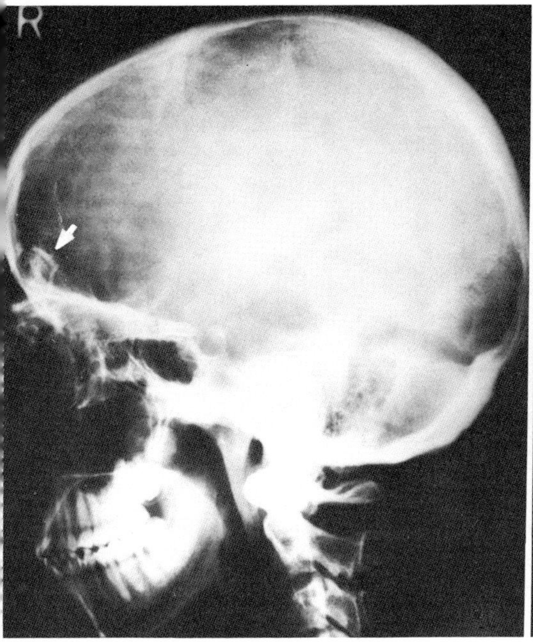

3/21B

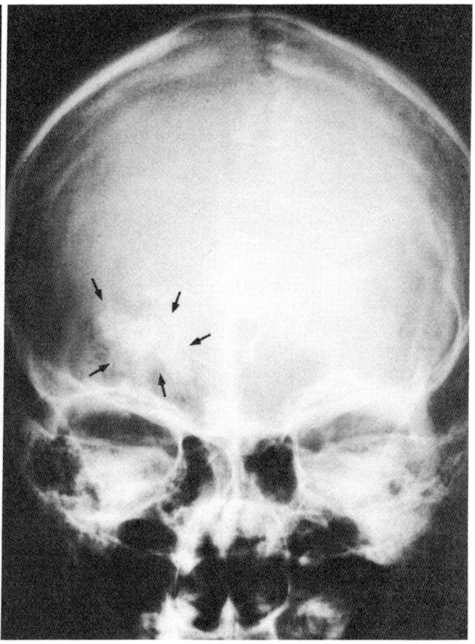

3/21C

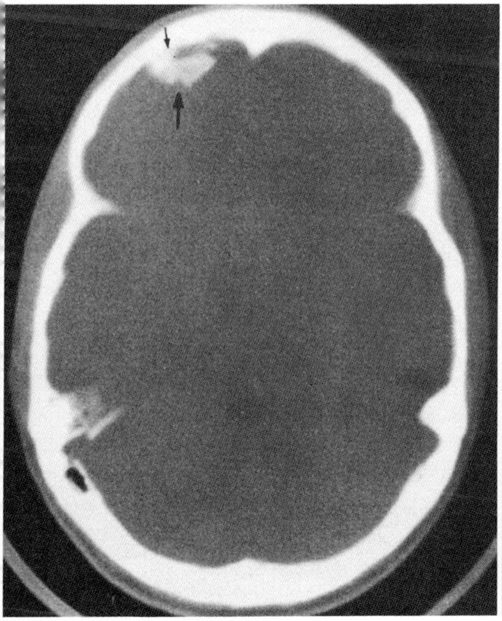

3/21D

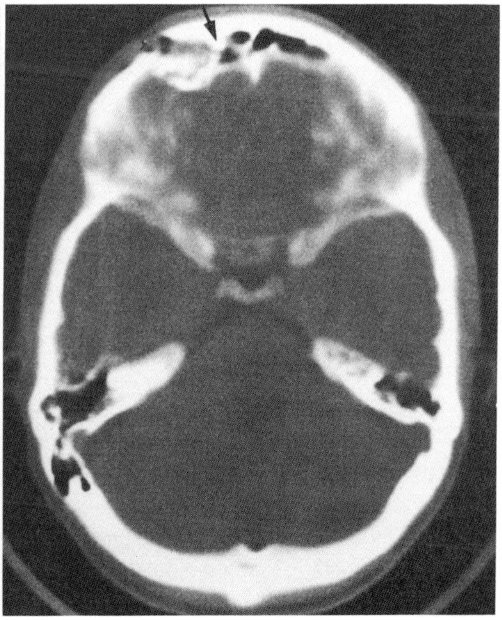

operation, local brain damage to the fracture fragments was found. No complications arose in the postoperative course. The patient was discharged 2 weeks later. Cranioplasty was necessary for the skull defect after a few months.

Slipping or Sliding

Case 13

Male, 13 years old. Because this boy strayed too far from the slope, he slipped off and tumbled more than 100 m over a rocky precipice, 30 m of it in a free fall. Upon hospital admission, the boy was comatose and had a dilated and fixed right pupil. Skull X-ray revealed a right temporoparietal fracture. Because of the neurological signs, a right craniotomy was performed immediately. An acute extensive subdural hematoma in the parietotemporal area was found and evacuated. Brain contusion with extensive brain swelling developed and called for aggressive surgical procedures, that is, craniectomy with opening of the dura and an open CSF drainage.

Case 14

Male, 30 years old. The patient slid off the ski slope and fell over a cliff, suffering a severe head injury. He was immediately brought to us by the helicopter rescue service. On admission the patient was drowsy and very restless with nasal bleeding and several bruises on the face, and moderately dilated pupils with prompt reaction to light. No paresis was found, nor were there neurological signs. Pulse 60/min, BP 130/90 mm Hg. Except for a bruise on the right thigh, there was no other injury to the body. In the course of about 30 min, the right pupil dilated slightly more than the left, for which reason an emergency right carotid arteriogram was performed. The AP view of the angiogram revealed a large avascular space in the right parietotemporal region and displacement of the anterior cerebral artery from right to left (fig. 3/22), and the weak visualization of the posterior part of the middle cerebral arteries (fig. 3/23) due to the epidural hematoma. At immediate

---

Fig. 3/22. Right anterior and middle cerebral arteries displaced leftward due to epidural hematoma. Extensive fracture in the right parietal area is also evident.

Fig. 3/23. Weak visualisation of posterior part of the middle cerebral arteries due to epidural hematoma.

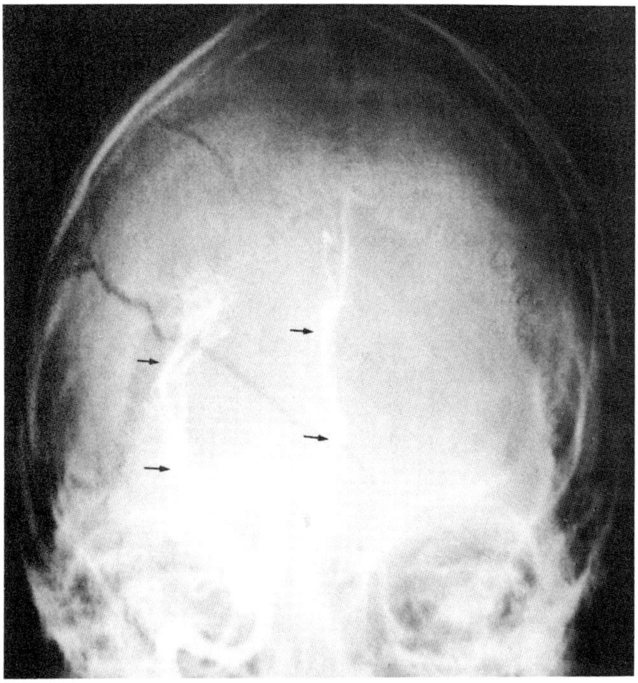

3/22

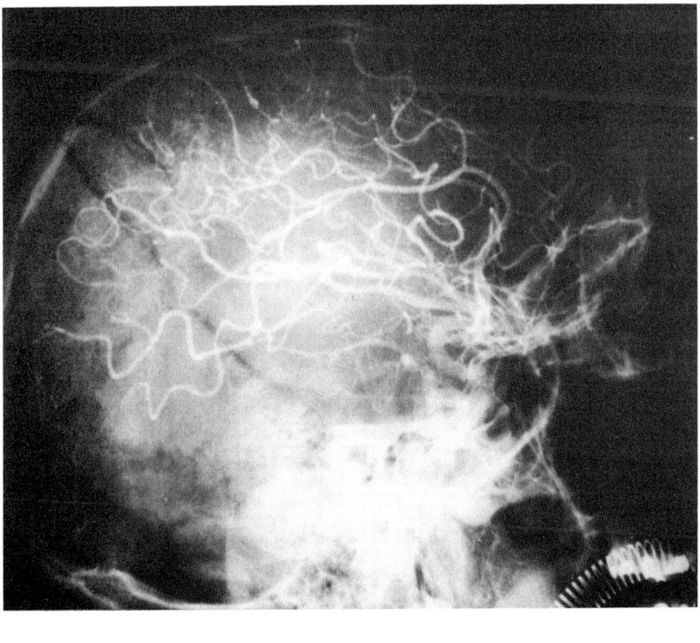

3/23

3/24

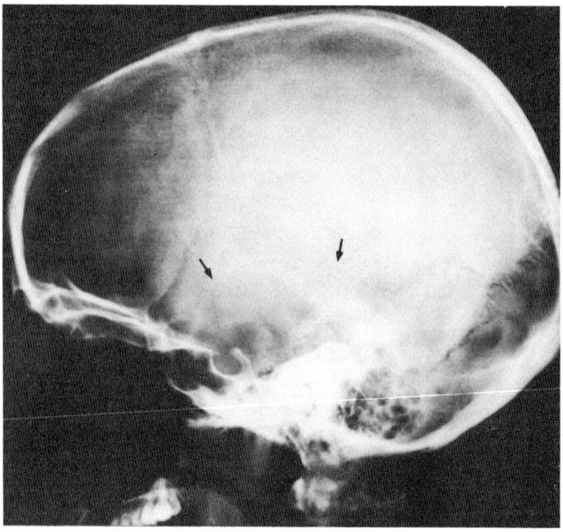

3/25

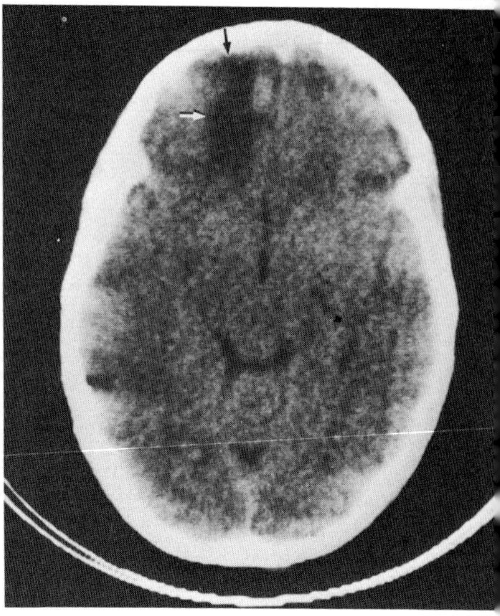

Fig. 3/24. Linear fracture in the right temporal region.
Fig. 3/25. CT scan showing the left frontal brain lesion after cerebral contusion.

craniotomy, an extensive epidural hematoma over the entire right cranium was evacuated. Furthermore, a depressed right temporobasal fracture with rupture of the dura was found, as well as subdural bleeding due to local brain laceration. He was intubated postoperatively and transferred to the intensive recovery ward. Postoperative progress was very satisfactory, so that the patient could be extubated on the 3rd day. The patient made a complete recovery.

Case 15

Female, 17 years old. The patient fell and slid on the open ski slope and then tumbled more than 10 m. She lost consciousness and was still unconscious 1 h later. Neurological finding showed pyramidal signs on the right. The skull X-ray revealed a right temporal fracture (fig. 3/24). CT scan revealed a brain lesion in the left frontal area (so-called contrecoup) (fig. 3/25). After about 2 weeks of conservative treatment she was discharged from hospital. She continued to suffer occasional headache. There was slight recovery of the lost sense of smell on the left.

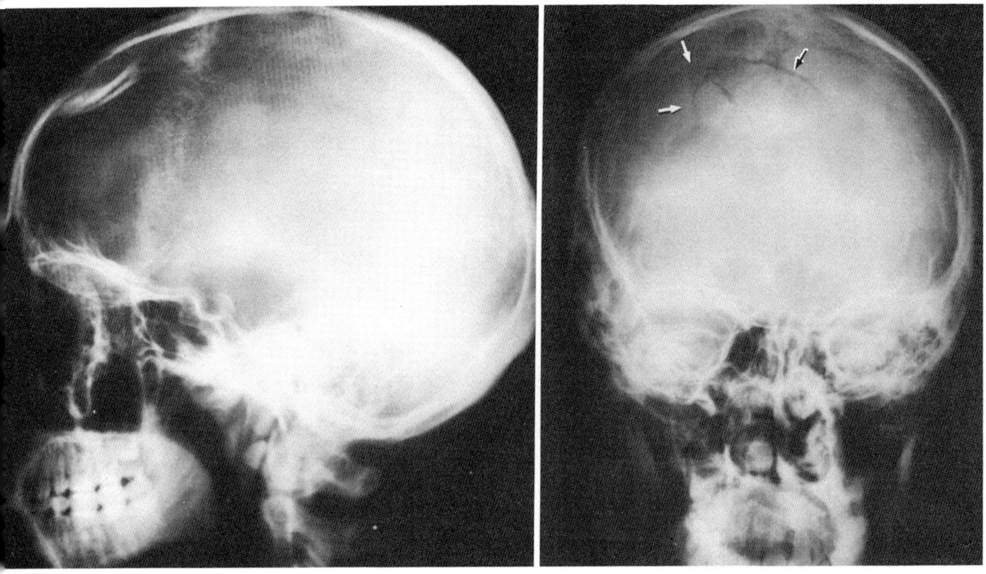

Fig. 3/26. Depressed fracture of mediofrontal region. **A** Lateral view. **B** AP view.

Hit by Ski-Lift

Case 16

Male, 13 years old. The patient received a blow to his head from a ski-lift T-bar. He was briefly unconscious and treated first by a local physician who sutured the open scalp wound in the left frontal region, he was then sent to our hospital. On admission, the patient's reactions were quite normal. He complained of frontal headache and nausea. During the neurological examination he vomited several times. Skull X-ray revealed a complete depressed fracture of the mediofrontal region (fig. 3/26A, B). As time went on, there was gradual deterioration in consciousness and he was finally deeply somnolent. The right pupil was dilated slightly. Immediate surgery to the open scalp wound and the depressed fracture revealed an epidural hematoma and many completely depressed bone fragments. Rupture of the dura mater and a brain contusion were also found. Careful debriding of all bone fragments, removal of epidural blood clots and repairing of the dura were performed. Antibiotics were administered to

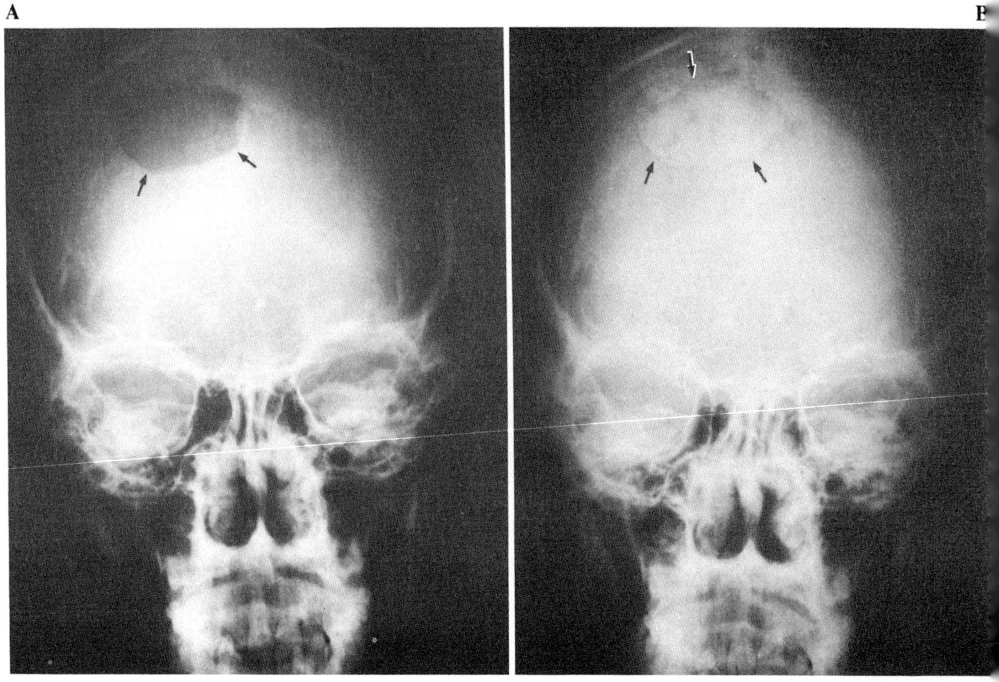

Fig. 3/27. A Bone defect. **B** Cranioplasty with Palacos.

prevent infection and antiedematous medication was also administered. The postoperative progress was good and the patient could be discharged without any symptoms 3 weeks later. The debrided bone defect (fig. 3/27A) was repaired 3 months later by Palacos cranioplasty (fig. 3/27B).

Case 17

Male, 15 years old. The patient suffered an open depressed skull fracture of the right parietal region from a blow by a ski-lift T-bar. He immediately lost consciousness and was brought to us as an emergency. On admission, the patient was conscious. There was an open laceration wound to the right parietal area of the scalp. The skull X-ray showed a bowl-shaped depressed fracture underneath the open scalp wound (fig. 3/28A, B). The open depressed fracture was operated at once. During the operation we found a ruptured dura and a small brain lesion. The skull defect was repaired by Palacos cranioplasty 3 months later (fig. 3/28C).

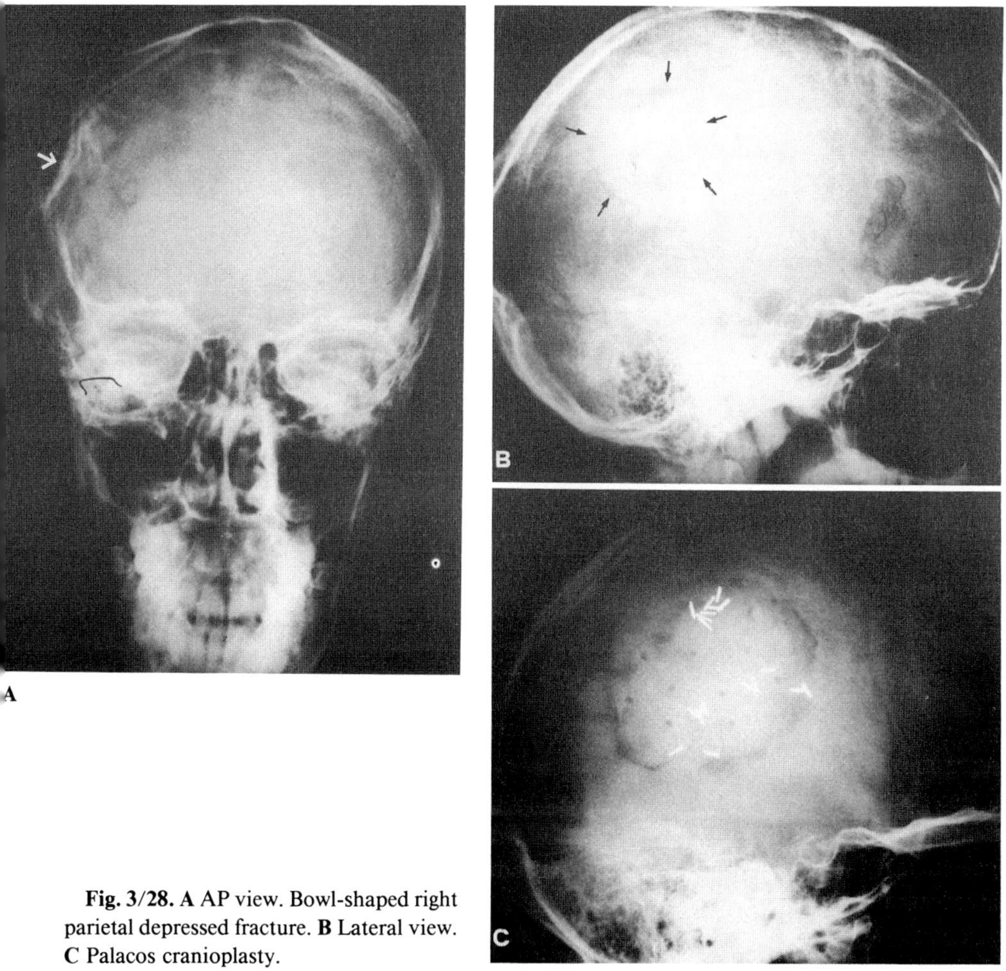

Fig. 3/28. A AP view. Bowl-shaped right parietal depressed fracture. **B** Lateral view. **C** Palacos cranioplasty.

Case 18

Female, 16 years old. She suffered an indirect head injury during the ride on the ski-lift. On the hard icy tracks, she fell due to loss of control and lost hold of the T-bar of the ski-lift. She slid downhill for about 300 m and her head hit the hard ski slope many times. The girl was found immediately in a comatose state. After intubation at the site of the accident, she was transferred to us by helicopter. In the emergency room, we found fixed

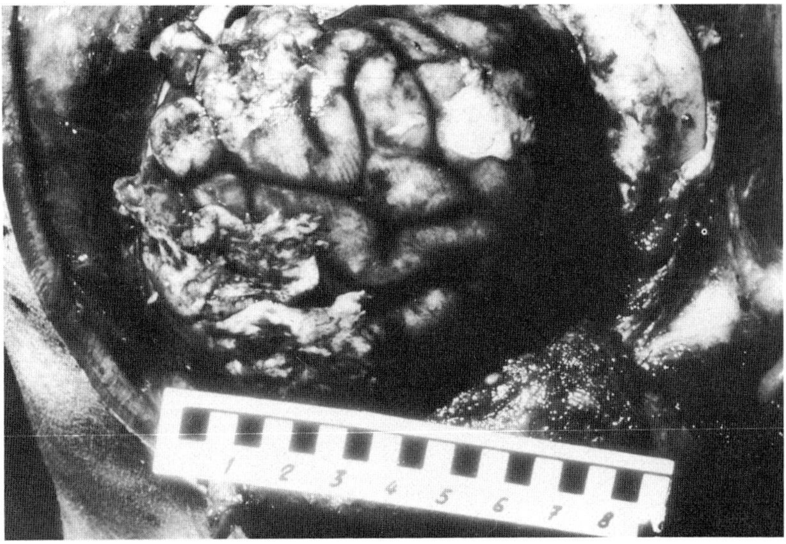

Fig. 3/29. Extensive brain contusion with herniation (finding during operation).

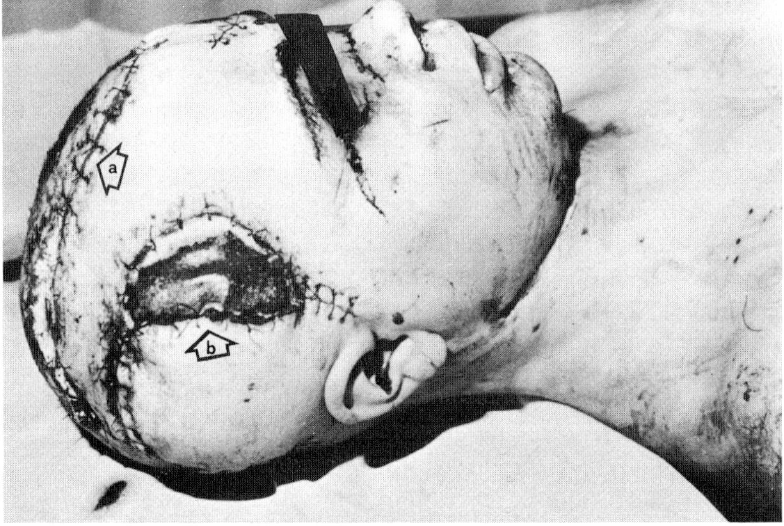

Fig. 3/30. Autopsy showed extensive brain damage in the right hemisphere.

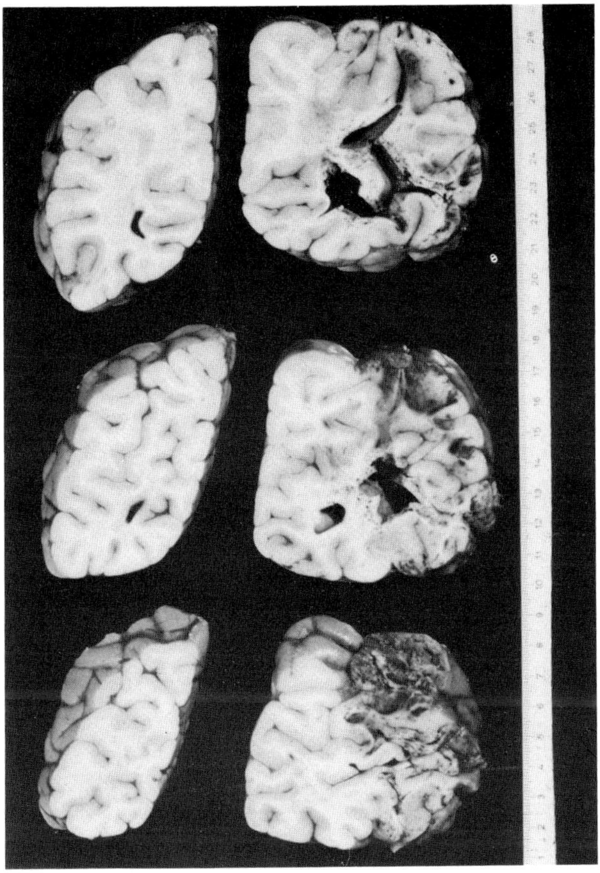

Fig. 3/31. Extensive damage to the right side of the brain (postmortem specimen).

dilated pupils with decerebrate rigidity on painful stimulation. Immediate decompressive right craniectomy was carried out. On opening the dura mater, herniation rapidly caused damage to the brain (fig. 3/29), even with mannitol infusion and hyperventilation. No skull fracture or epidural hematoma was found. The patient died shortly after the decompressive operation (fig. 3/30). Autopsy showed the extensive contusion on the right hemisphere with extensive edematous swelling (fig. 3/31). This accident caused a fatal indirect head injury.

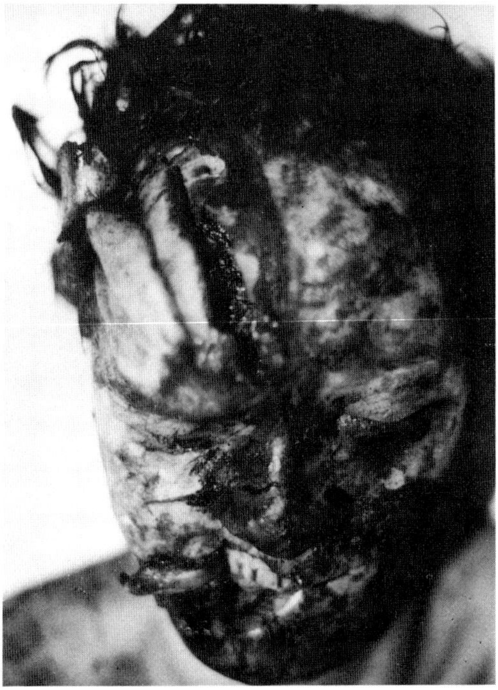

Fig. 3/32. Severe head injury.

Collision with Various Obstacles

Case 19: Wooden Railings

Male, 28 years old. The man, skiing at high speed in good weather and on powder snow, lost his balance on a smooth, straight and wide slope shortly before a wooden bridge, where there was a fence about 15 m long and 1.5 m high. As a result he slid head-first into the wooden bridge railings. The patient suffered very severe head injuries which caused his death at the site of the accident.

Case 20: Boulder

Male, 40 years old. While skiing on a well-prepared slope in good weather and snow conditions, he left the slope and crashed, his head hitting a boulder. The patient immediately became comatose. In spite of very prompt rescue by helicopter, the patient died during the flight as a result of

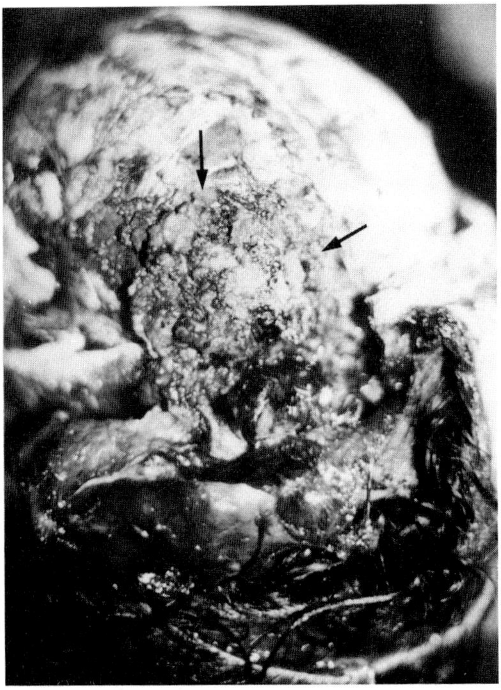

Fig. 3/33. Picture taken with scalp peeled forward. Much grit in the epidural area.

his severe head injury. Externally, an extensive compound, comminuted, depressed right frontoparietal fracture was found, together with extensive deep lacerations of the whole right side of face and a torn tongue (fig. 3/32). During the postmortem examination, a large quantity of grit was found in the right frontal epidural area under the extensive open scalp laceration (fig. 3/33) and extensive skull fracture (fig. 3/34), as well as extensive brain damage in the right hemisphere (fig. 3/35).

Case 21: Rock

Male, 21 years old. The patient went skiing on fresh snow with 4 friends. He fell over a rock hidden by show and suffered an open head injury. On hospital admission, the patient complained of headache and nausea but there was no disturbance of consciousness. No neurological signs were found. There was a small open scalp laceration in the right frontotemporal region. The skull X-ray showed a depressed fracture just under

3/34

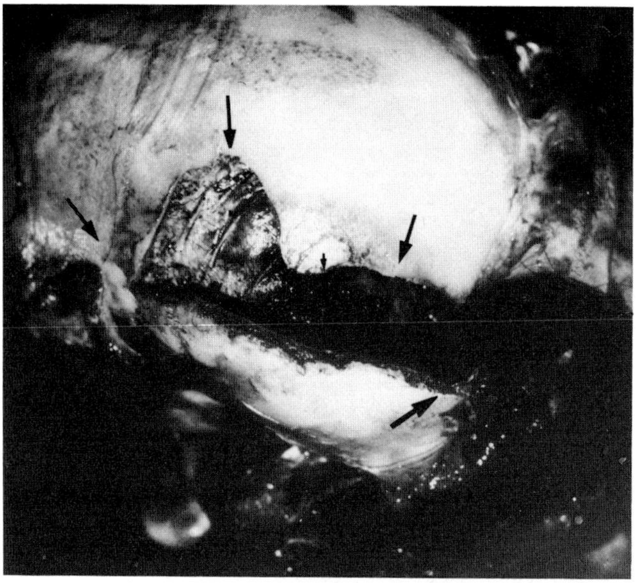

3/35

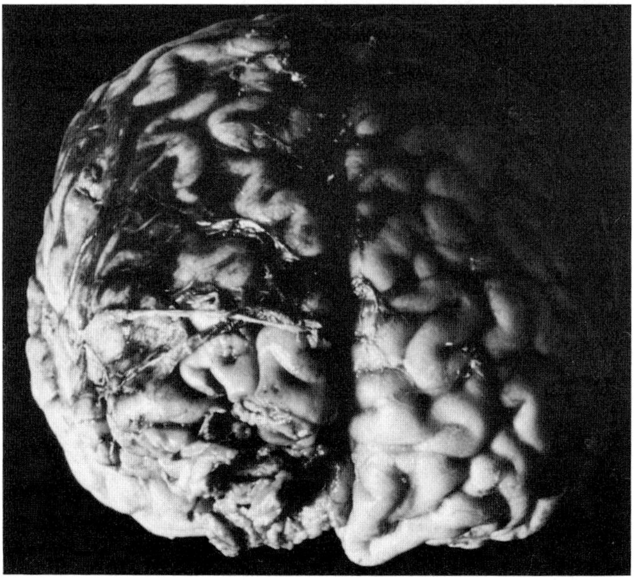

Fig. 3/34. Severe open right compound, comminuted, depressed fracture in the frontoparietal area with extensive brain laceration.

Fig. 3/35. Extensive brain contusion-laceration in the right hemisphere.

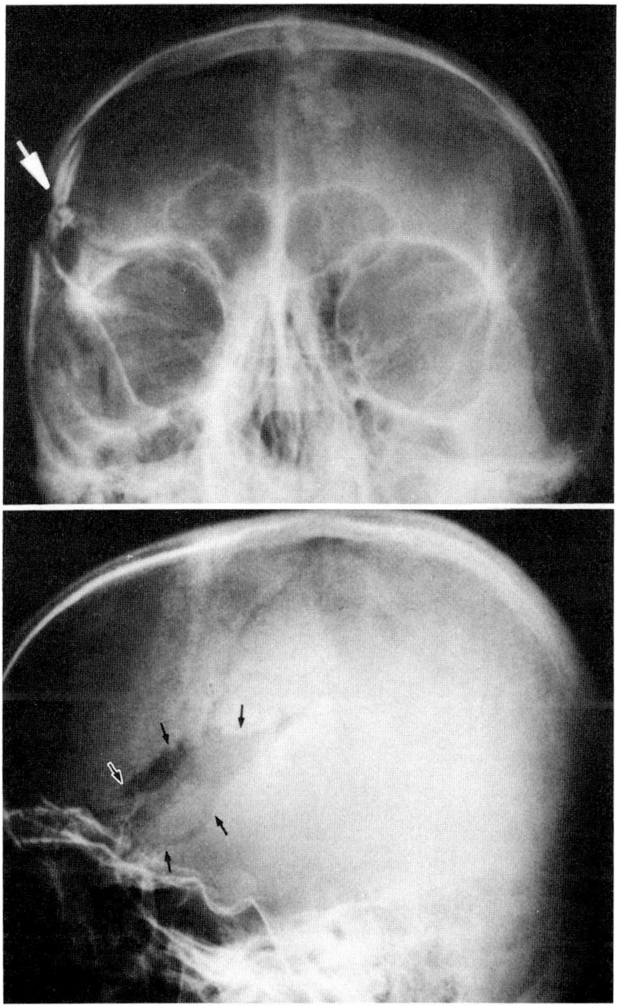

A

B

Fig. 3/36. Right open depressed fracture in the temporal area. **A** AP view. **B** Lateral view.

the scalp wound (fig. 3/36A, B). Immediate surgery was performed on the open depressed skull fracture. The fragments of bone were removed. The lacerated dura and local brain damage was observed. The necrotic brain tissues were removed and the dural laceration was closed with lyophilized dura.

Case 22: Rock

Male, 12 years old. The patient fell on the slope and slid off toward the right, hitting his head violently on a rock. The boy immediately lost consciousness and he was transferred to us by helicopter. On admission the child was stuporous. In the medioparietal region there was an extensive open laceration to the scalp, and a depressed fracture was palpable. The right pupil was slightly dilated with slow reaction to light. BP 120/90 mm Hg, pulse 132/min. X-rays of the skull showed a compound, comminuted, depressed medioparietal fracture and frontal pneumocephalus (fig. 3/37, 3/38). The open depressed fracture had to be treated surgically at once. Rupture of the dura and damage to the sagittal sinus with bleeding were found and repaired. The child complained of recurrent backade. X-rays of the thoracic spine revealed a compressed fracture (T-6) without luxation. The patient was discharged after 4 weeks of postoperative care in generally good condition. The extensive bone defect was covered with Palacos material in a second surgical procedure a few months later.

Case 23: Rock

Male, 20 years old. The patient was skiing on fresh snow when he fell. Both skis were released automatically, and the patient was thrown, hitting his head against a rock. He showed retrograde amnesia. No neurological disorders were found. There was a left frontal scalp laceration. Skull X-ray revealed a fracture of the lateral lower orbital ridge, extending to the left maxilla (fig. 3/39). CT scan showed fracture of the nasal ethmoid complex on the left, and the maxilla and zygomatic bone were slightly displaced (fig. 3/40). The fracture was treated conservatively at first. The further course was excellent and without complication, and 3 weeks later he could be discharged. Later, the patient noticed an occasional discharge in his left nostril, most likely due to a leakage of CSF. The nasal fluid was examined. It contained sugar. The CSF fistula is shown in figure 3/40. This loss of cerebrospinal fluid was repaired by bifrontal craniotomy (with duraplasty).

Case 24: Ski-Lift Mast

Male, 36 years old. The patient fell one afternoon, crashing his head against a ski-lift mast. He immediately lost consciousness. First aid was provided at the local hospital, and then he was transported to us for emergency surgical treatment of the open depressed fracture. On admission to our department the patient showed inadequate response to painful stimuli bilaterally. There was a diagonal open left frontal scalp wound with pro-

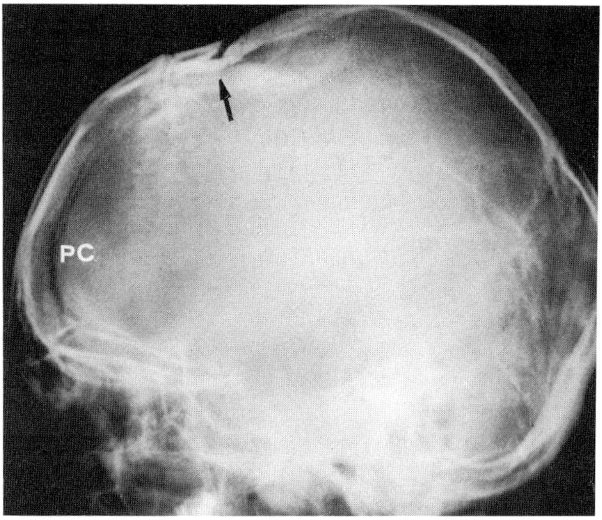

3/37

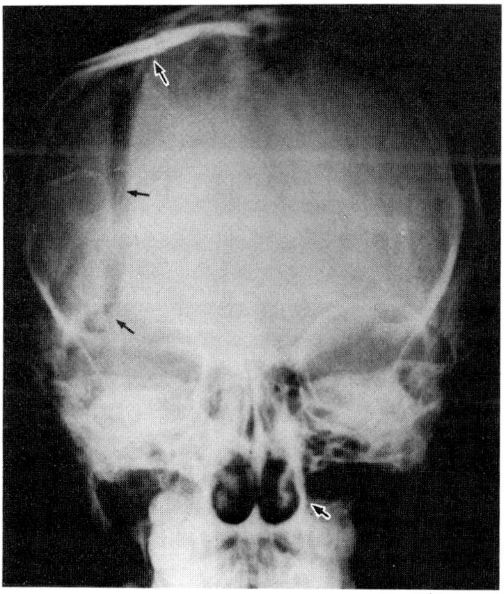

3/38

Fig. 3/37. Medioparietal compound, comminuted, depressed fracture with frontal pneumocephalus (PC).

Fig. 3/38. AP view. Large compound, comminuted, depressed fracture.

3/39
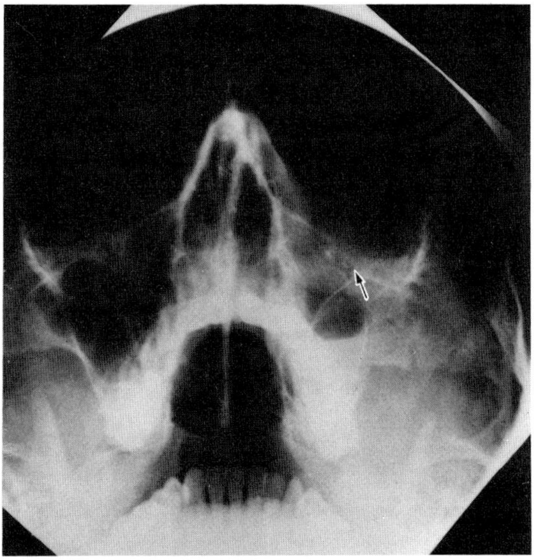

3/40
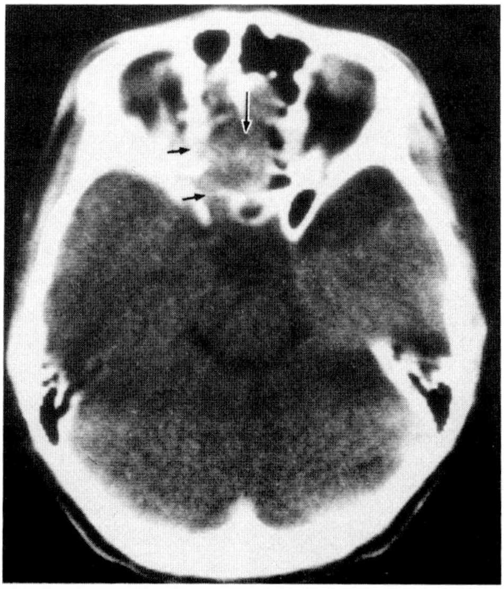

Fig. 3/39. Base of left orbital fracture slightly displaced.
Fig. 3/40. Fracture of the left nasal ethmoid with CSF fistula.

3/41A

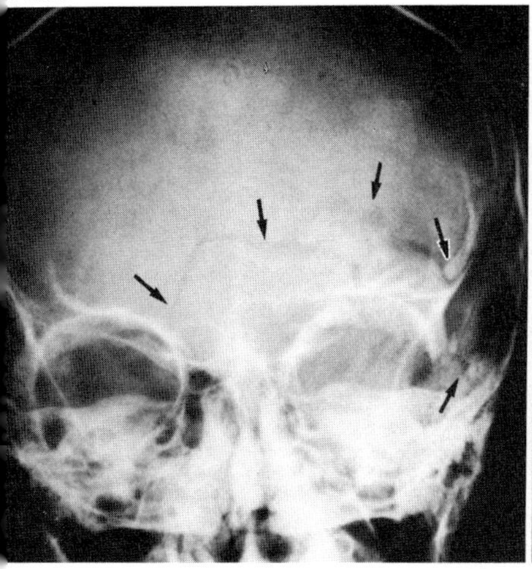

3/41B

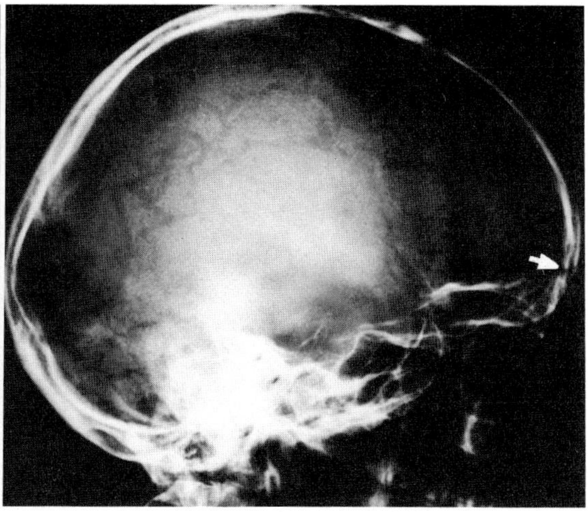

3/42A

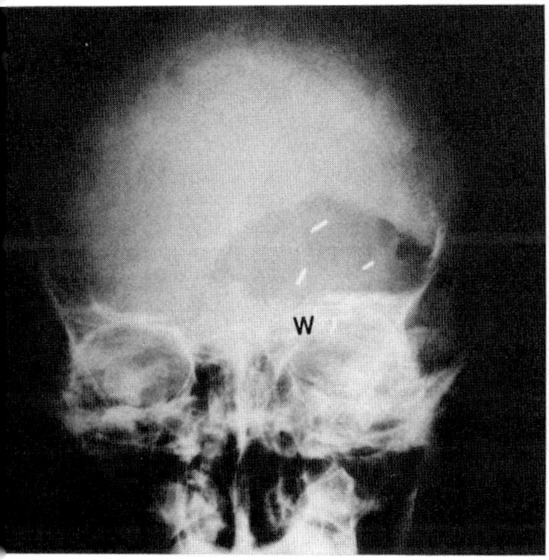

3/42B

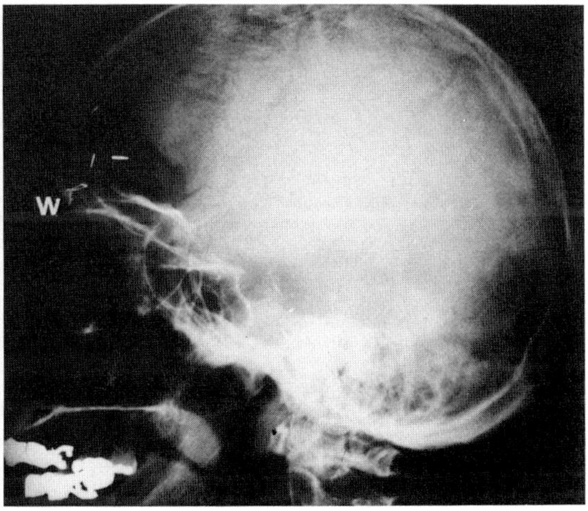

Fig. 3/41. A AP view. **B** Lateral view. Left frontal depressed fracture with linear fracture extending over the right frontal area.

Fig. 3/42A, B. Postoperative. Bone defect and fixed wire (W).

nounced eyelid hematoma. No neurological disorders were found. X-rays of the skull revealed a depressed fracture over the left orbit and a fracture of the lateral roof of the orbit extending to the zygomatic attachment. The orbital fracture was displaced slightly downward and backward, and there was also a linear fracture over the right frontal area (fig. 3/41A, B). Imme-

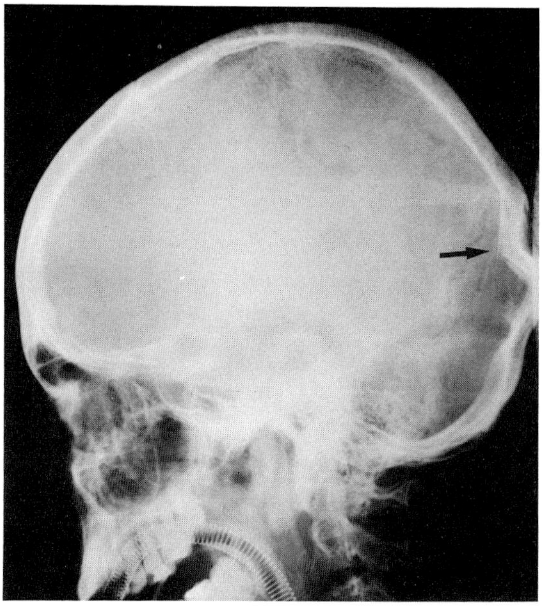

Fig. 3/43. Occipital depressed fracture.

diate surgery was carried out. In particular, the fractured lateral roof of the orbit was debrided and the displaced orbital ridge was fixed with wire after repositioning (fig. 3/42A, B). The wide rupture of the dura mater underneath the depressed fracture and the damage to the brain were also cleaned up. His recovery was complete within 3 weeks of injury. A bone defect repair by Palacos cranioplasty was performed about 3 months later in his home country (FRG).

Case 25: Stone

Male, 15 years old. The patient lost control while skiing fast, fell on the slope and rolled over many times. During this, his head hit the ground and then stone, and he suffered an open occipital depressed skull fracture (fig. 3/43). The patient vomited many times during transportation to the hospital. He was drowsy. He responded to pain stimulation with motor coordination and spontaneous pyramidal signs. Near the external occipital protuberance a large scalp wound was found and the depressed fracture was palpable under the wound. It was possible to reposition the open depressed fracture perfectly. No postoperative complications were observed.

A

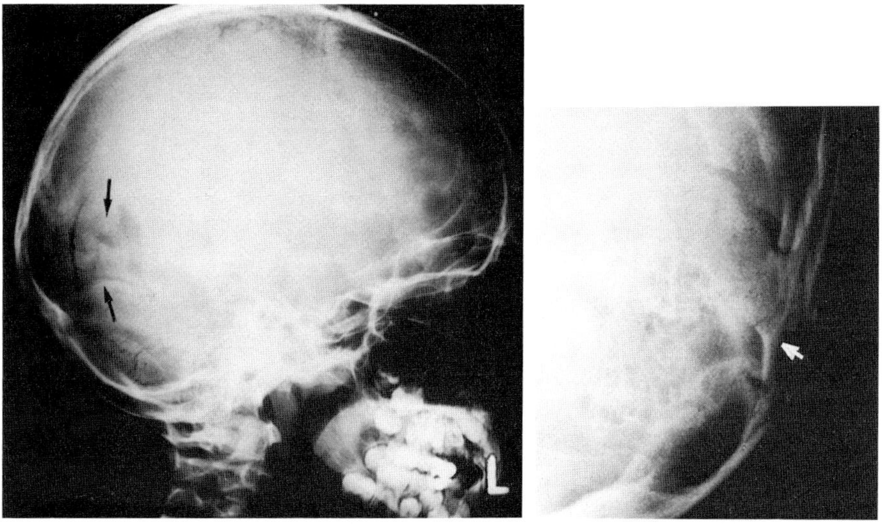

B

Fig. 3/44. **A** Left occipital depressed fracture (lateral view). **B** Illustration of the depressed fracture in oblique view.

Case 26: Stone

Male, 10 years old. Skiing carelessly and at high speed, he lost control and fell on the open slope. His head crashed against the slope which had insufficient snow (stony ground), and he suffered an open left occipital depressed fracture, with amnesia about the cause of the accident. The patient vomited many times. Skull X-ray revealed a left occipital depressed fracture (fig. 3/44A, B). This closed depressed fracture was repaired 5 days later by surgical repositioning. No postoperative complications were observed.

Case 27: Base of Pole

Male, 12 years old. The patient fell on the open ski slope and then slid off, hitting his head against the concrete base of a pole. After the accident he was somnolent for a few hours. Neurological examination findings were normal. On the head there was a large laceration of the left parietal area of the scalp. Skull X-ray showed a depressed fracture in the area of the scalp wound (fig. 3/45). This open depressed fracture was immediately treated by surgery. Laceration of the dura, but no brain damage was found. The post-

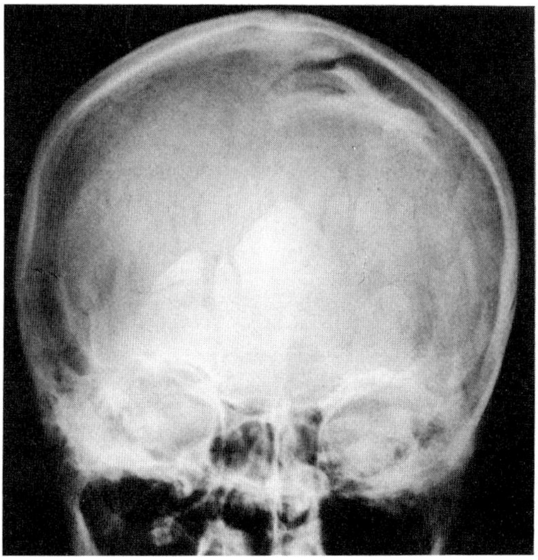

Fig. 3/45. Left parietal depressed skull fracture.

operative course was good and the patient was discharged symptom-free after 12 days. The bone defect was repaired 3 months later by Palacos cranioplasty.

Case 28: Tree

Female, 11 years old. The girl crashed head-on into a tree on a forest path. She was unconscious and was first taken to the district hospital. There they found an open depressed fracture in the left frontotemporal region (fig. 3/46A, B). She was transferred to our hospital for operative treatment. The patient was alert and oriented. Neurological examination findings were normal. It was possible to reposition the depressed fracture perfectly. The patient made a complete recovery.

Case 29: Ski Rack

Male, 17 years old. According to eye witnesses, the young man crashed into a ski rack. After the accident, he was unconscious and vomited many times. After emergency transfer to the local hospital, a right frontal scalp laceration was treated. His right pupil was slightly larger than the left. Spon-

3/46A

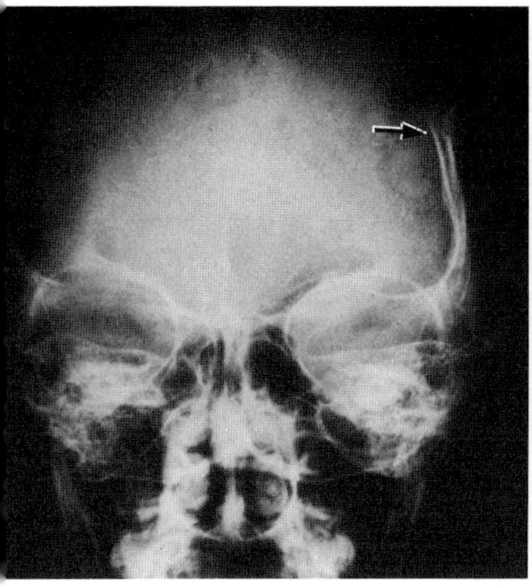

3/46B

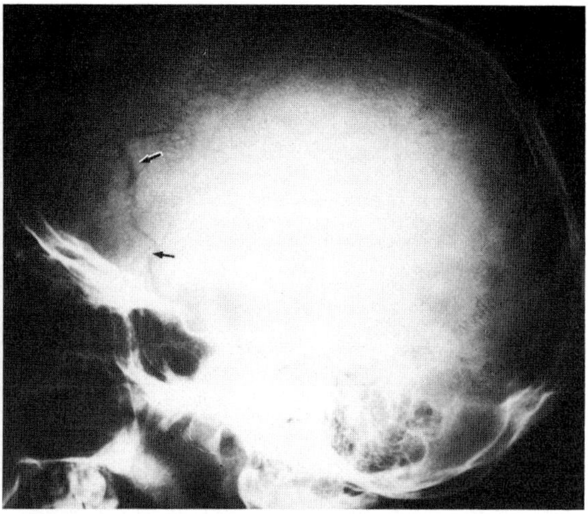

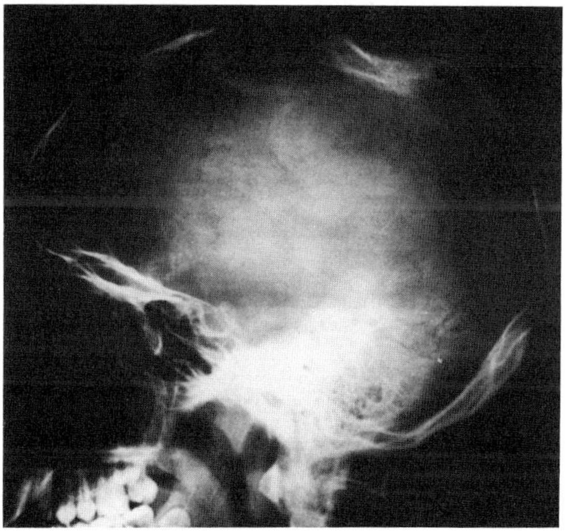

3/47

Fig. 3/46. Left open depressed fracture in the frontotemporal area. **A** AP and **B** lateral view.

Fig. 3/47. Depressed right paramedian parietal fracture.

taneous restlessness appeared and progressed until the patient lapsed into deep unconsciousness. In addition, a huge eyelid swelling and petechial hemorrhage developed on the right. Skull X-ray showed a paramedian parietal depressed fracture (fig. 3/47). Because of the possibility of intracranial hemorrhage underneath the fracture, the patient was transferred to us as an

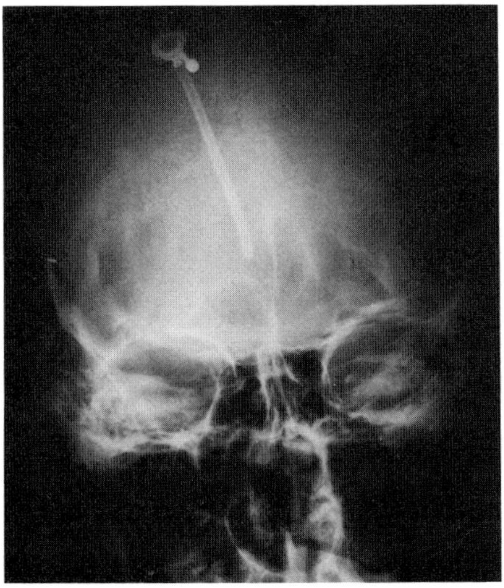

Fig. 3/48. Large parietotemporal decompressive craniectomy and ventricular CSF drainage.

emergency. On admission, he responded to pain stimuli only on the right. The right pupil was moderately dilated and fixed. The left pupil was narrowed with prompt reaction to light. A left central facial paresis and bilateral Babinski signs were found. During operation a large subdural hematoma was found and removed. There was a diffuse subdural brain contusion. Because of malignant brain edema due to diffuse brain damage, the dura was not closed and a ventricular CSF-drain was inserted (fig. 3/48). In addition, a large decompressive craniectomy was performed and artificial respiration maintained with intubation. The postoperative progress was slow but very satisfactory. 6 days later the patient was awake and responsive. He still had left facial paresis and left hemiparesis. The subsequent postoperative course was very good. Because of the left hemiparesis intensive daily physiotherapy was performed. 4 weeks later, he was transferred to a hospital near his home for continuation of physical treatment.

Case 30: Hut Wall

Male, 53 years old. Skiing along a narrow path to another ski slope, the patient crashed straight into the concrete wall of the mountain hut, hitting his head violently. The skier immediately lost consciousness. He was in a

A B

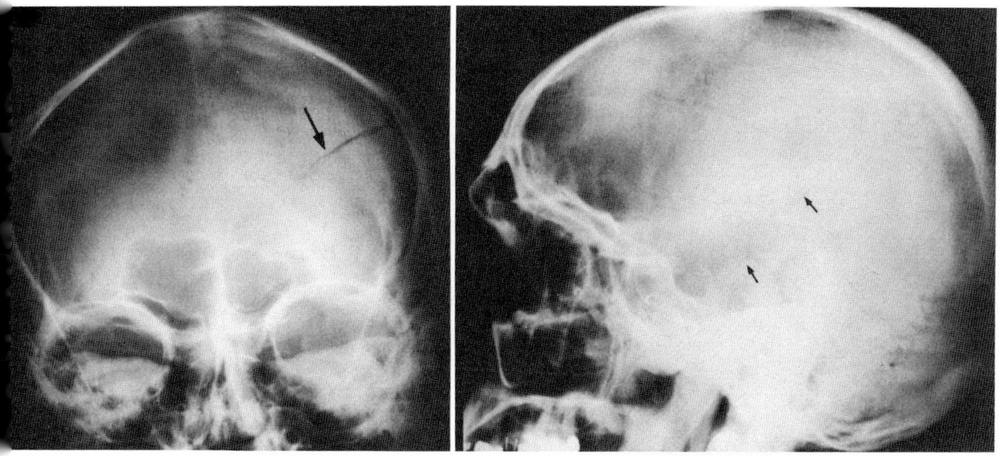

Fig. 3/49. Left linear parietal fracture. **A** AP view. **B** Lateral view.

stupor and spontaneously restless. He responded to pain stimulation with good motor coordination. Both pyramidal signs were present. No other lesion except the head injury was found. The skull X-ray showed an extensive linear fracture in the left parietal region (fig. 3/49A, B). A few days later he complained of left chest pains. Chest X-ray showed a left costal fracture. With conservative treatment he was able 3 days later to answer questions coherently. After 3 weeks he was discharged from hospital in good general condition.

Case 31: Snow Plough

Female, 16 years old. Fell on the ski slope and by parked tanker strangulated her head completely. She was found later unconscious and with respiratory arrest. Artificial respiration and intubation were immediately applied and she was transferred to us by helicopter. In the emergency room, she was found to be in a state of coma with contracted pupils, and extensive petechial swelling of face and eyes (fig. 3/50). A CT scan of the head revealed diffuse brain congestion (fig. 3/51A, B), but no brain contusion or hemorrhage. Intracranial pressure monitoring (ICPM) with measurements via an epidural screw were carried out and initially showed about 25 mm Hg ICP. With antiedematous medication and artificial respiration, she regained consciousness 24 h later. 4 days later she was transferred to a hospital at home in Germany at her family's request.

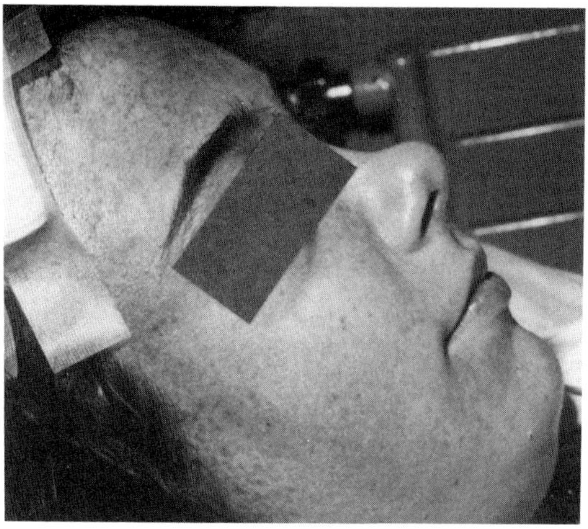

Fig. 3/50. Extensive petechial swelling of face and eyes.

A

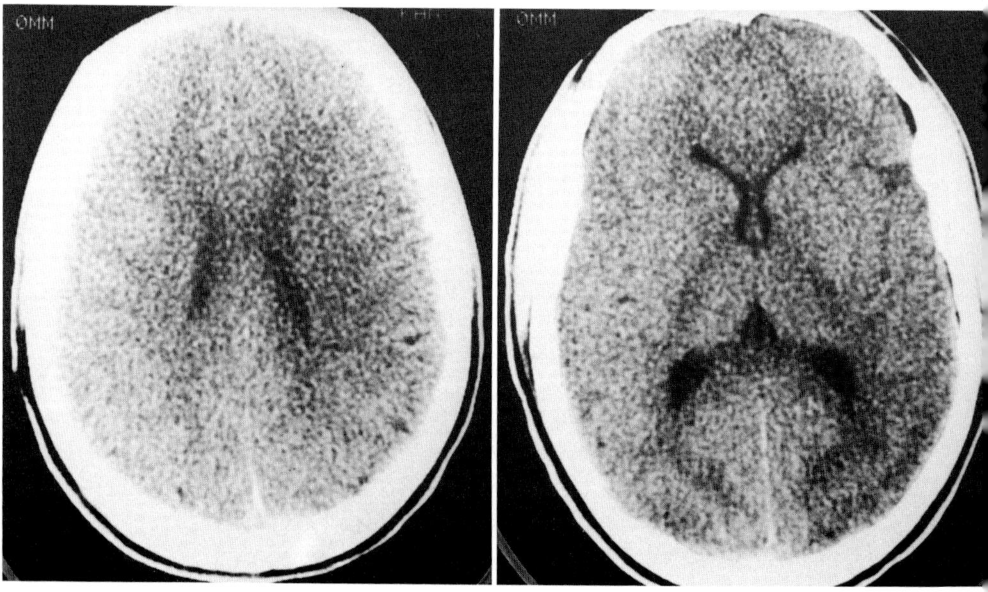

Fig. 3/51 A, B. Extensive brain swelling with no lesions.

3/52

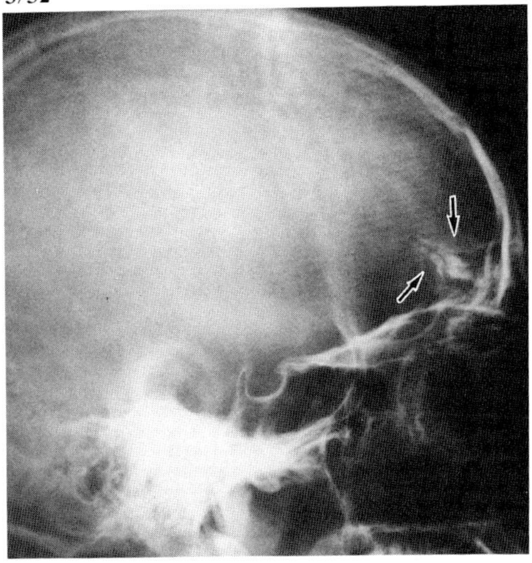

3/53

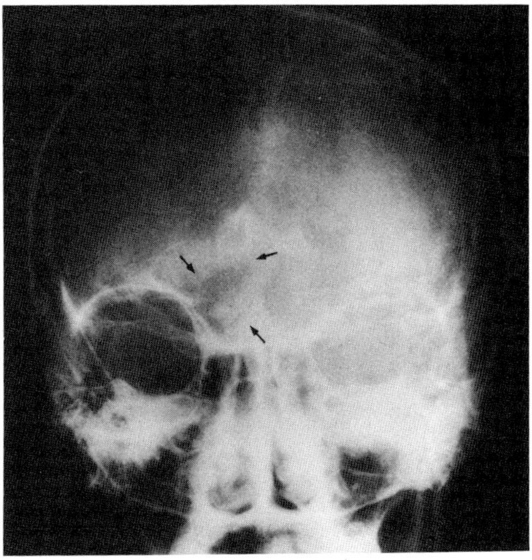

Fig. 3/52. Right frontal depressed skull fracture.
Fig. 3/53. Depressed fracture of the right frontal sinus.

Unknown Causes

Case 32

Male, 30 years old. The patient came from Germany. He was found unconscious beside the ski slope. The reason for the accident is unknown. He was transported by helicopter to us. On admission, he was somnolent, with an open scalp laceration in the right frontal region. Neurological examination findings normal. Skull X-ray revealed a depressed fracture in the area of the right frontal sinus (fig. 3/52, 3/53). During the immediate surgery on the depressed fracture, we found dural laceration with brain damage. An unstable orbital fracture was fixed with wire and necrotic brain tissue beneath the depressed fracture was carefully debrided (fig. 3/54). Open frontal sinus fracture was closed with Palacos material and lyophilized dura.

Case 33

Male, 20 years old. The skier was found in an unconscious state one morning near the slope. During first aid at the hospital after transport by rescue helicopter, a right brain stem syndrome was found, also the right

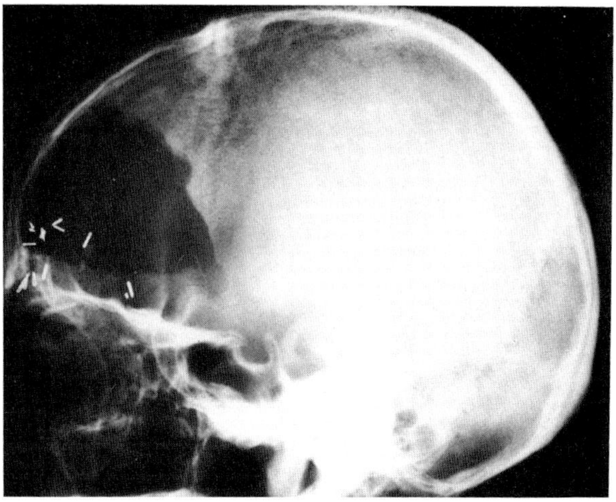

Fig. 3/54. Bone defect after surgical treatment of the depressed fracture.

pupil was dilated and fixed. His condition was comatose with irregular respiration and unstable circulatory reactions (hypertension and tachycardia). Reacted to painful stimuli with decerebrate postures. Furthermore, otorrhea on the right was seen. Skull X-ray showed an extensive left occipitoparietal fracture (fig. 3/55A, B). The computed tomogram revealed a left parieto-occipital epidural hematoma (fig. 3/56). Immediate craniectomy and removal of the hematoma were performed. Despite immediate surgical treatment, the brain stem symptoms persisted and the patient died a few days later.

Case 34

Male, 14 years old. The patient suffered an accident of unknown cause. He was transported to us by helicopter. He was confused and agitated. The pupils reacted normally and no hemiparesis was found. Bilateral Babinski signs. Abdomen was slightly tender with shock reactions. Immediate laparotomy was carried out. Intraabdominal bleeding from rupture of the liver was found. Slow and progressive deterioration from consciousness to coma, and 2 days later the right pupil abruptly became dilated and fixed. Angiogram showed space-occupying shadows in the right temporo-occipital region. Craniectomy was performed. Extensive hemorrhagic, necrotic brain damage and edema were found, and aggressive decompressive procedures

A B

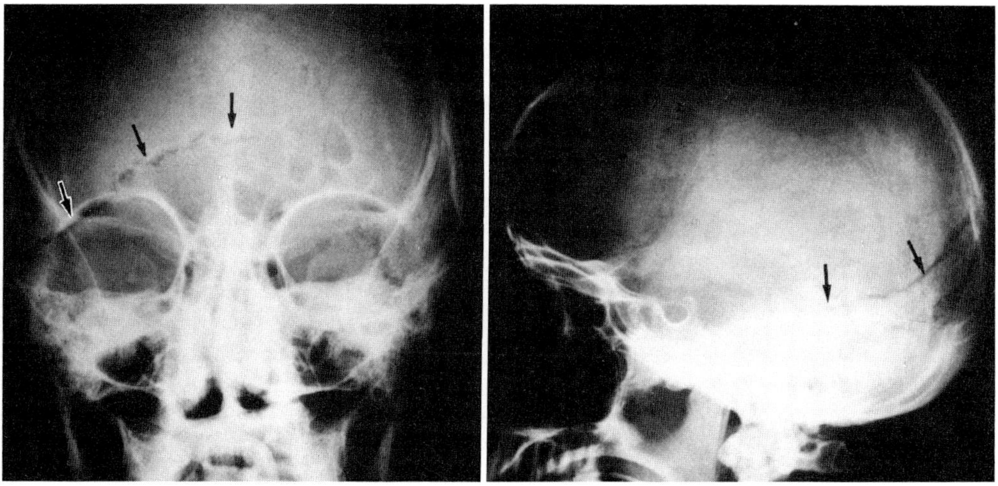

Fig. 3/55 A, B. AP and lateral view. Extensive left linear fracture in the parieto-occipital region.

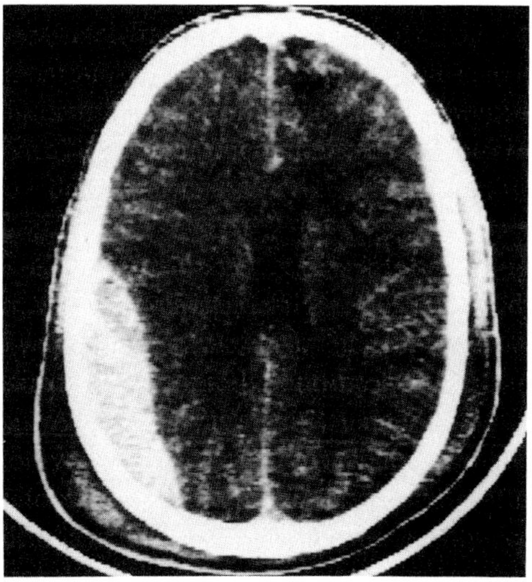

Fig. 3/56. CT scan. Epidural hematoma under the linear fracture in the left parieto-occipital region.

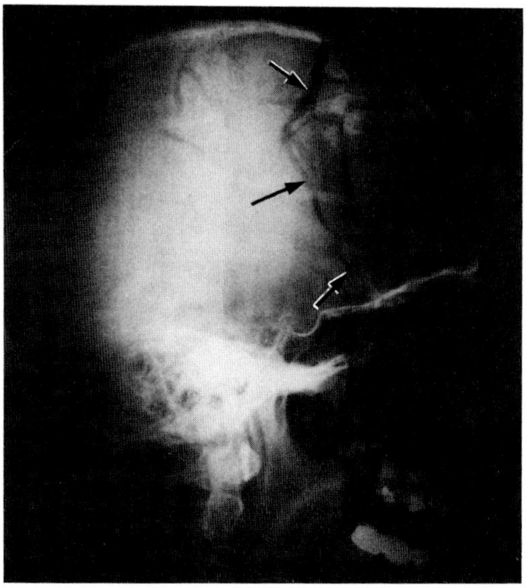

Fig. 3/57. Compound, comminuted, depressed fracture in the right frontal region.

applied. After the operation the brain stem syndrome disappeared completely. 4 days later the right pupil again abruptly became dilated and fixed. Repeat craniectomy showed extensive brain herniation due to extensive edematous reactions. The patient was comatose for more than 2 weeks and then a tracheotomy was performed. Despite intensive care, his condition progressively worsened, and 2 months later he died from central respiratory and cardiac arrest due to severe brain contusion.

Case 35

Male, 14 years old. The patient hit his head directly (cause unknown). On admission he was comatose. Right frontal an approximately 7-cm-long scalp laceration was found. Skull X-ray showed a compound, comminuted, depressed fracture in the right frontal area extending to the median line (fig. 3/57). During operation, an extensive depressed fracture and diverse linear fractures extending frontobasal on the right were discovered. Displaced fractures of the right orbital roof and rupture of the dura mater with brain contusion under the depressed fracture and damage of the superior sagittal sinus were also found.

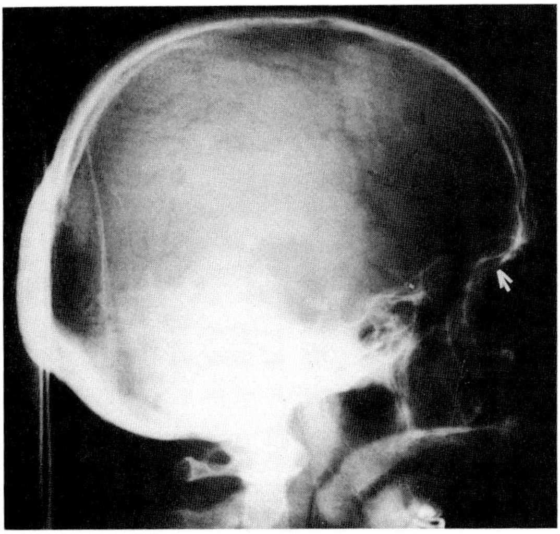

Fig. 3/58. Fracture of the nasal bone and frontobasal fracture.

Alcohol

Case 36

Male, 23 years old. The patient was skiing under the influence of alcohol when he tumbled over a wall about 3 m high and finished up in a garden fence. He immediately lost consciousness. On admission to hospital the patient was somnolent with alcohol on his breath. Skull X-ray revealed a frontobasal fracture and a fracture of the nasal bone (fig. 3/58).

Combined Injuries (Head and Neck)

Case 37

Male, 36 years old. The patient is in charge of rescues at the slope complex at Flims. During an inspection trip in January 1979, he collided with a telegraph pole hitting his head violently. According to his statement he was unconscious for more than an hour. He was able to call for help using

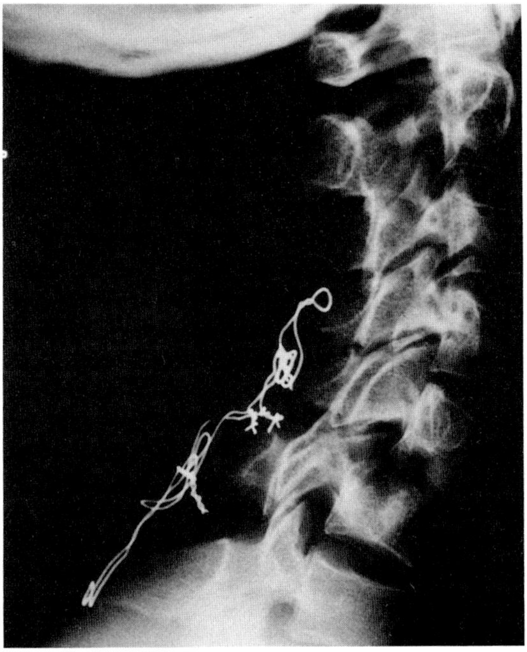

Fig. 3/59. Anterior-posterior fixation.

his own radio, and was transported by sled to the valley and by helicopter to our neurosurgical department. On arrival, the patient complained of severe pain in the cervical region and the head. The patient was in poor general condition. Fully aware of time, place and surroundings. A large right-hemisphere laceration wound to scalp, and pressure pain above the vertebrae from C4 to C7 with pronounced hard spasm of the neck muscles were found. The left forearm and hand were distinctly weaker than the right. Left biceps-tendon reflexes clearly weaker than the right. Hypesthesia and hypalgesia in the left C6 dermatome. No pyramidal signs. The cervical spine X-ray revealed a fracture-dislocation C5/6. After dressing the large laceration wound on the head, a head/skeletal tongs traction was applied. The patient subsequently recuperated rather well and the neurological signs slowly disappeared. After reduction of the fracture-dislocation, surgery was performed (fig. 3/59), i.e. posterior wire fixation of the C4 to C7 spinal process and anterior spondylodesis C5/6 by the Cloward method. Postoperative recovery was completely without complications. The patient could

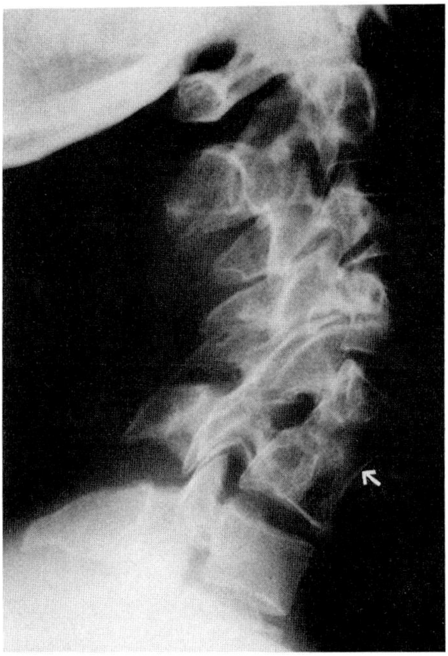

Fig. 3/60. Good fusion C5/C6 and wire removed.

be sent home in good general condition 3 weeks later, without any neurological deficits. The wire in the posterior region was removed 9 months later (fig. 3/60).

Case 38

Male, 16 years old. The patient fell and collided with stone objects at the side of the ski slope. He was conscious on admission. Right hemiparesis and sensory disturbance at the C5 dermatome on the right were found. Skull X-rays showed a left parietal open depressed fracture (fig. 3/61A, B) and dislocation C4 and C5 with stretching of the spine (fig. 3/62A). The open depressed skull fracture underwent immediate surgery. Subsequently, a skeletal caliper traction was also applied. Cervical spine subluxation was treated 10 days later by anterior spondylodesis C4/5 by the method of Cloward (fig. 3/62B). 3 weeks later the patient was sent home in good general condition. The left parietal skull defect was treated 3 months later by Palacos cranioplasty (fig. 3/63).

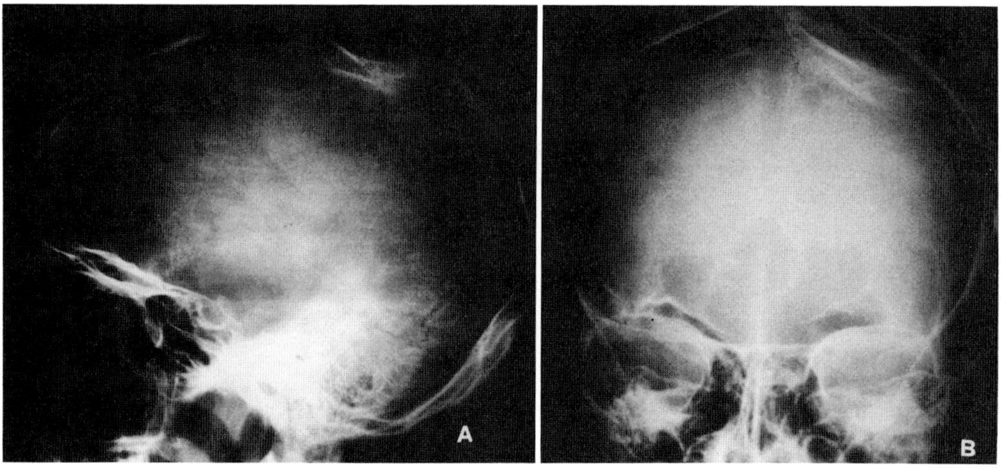

Fig. 3/61A, B. Left parietal depressed fracture.

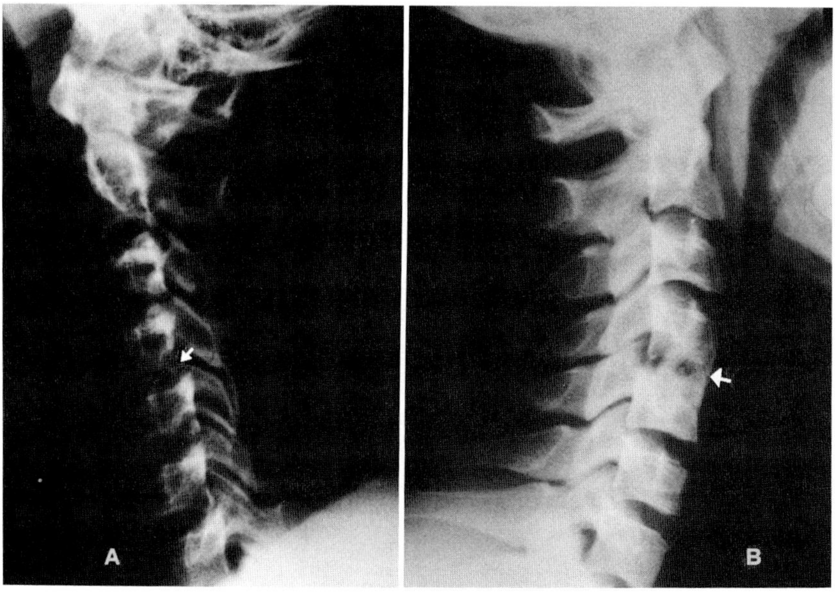

Fig. 3/62. Subluxation C4/5 with stretching of the spine (**A**), and anterior spondylodesis (**B**).

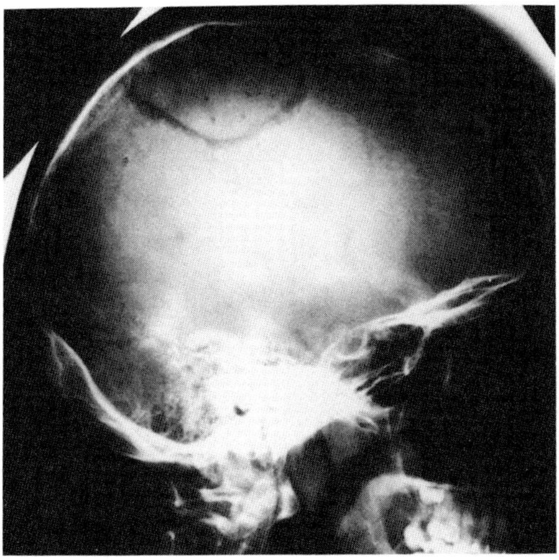

Fig. 3/63. Skull defect with Palacos cranioplasty.

Statistical Data

All patients came from the canton of Graubünden where the largest winter sport resorts in Switzerland are located. A total of 638 patients (fig. 3/64) with head injuries were treated from 1974 to 1982 (8 years), 283 of these cases in the hospitals of Davos (81), Samedan (75), Savognin (76) and Arosa (51) between 1974 and 1978. 355 patients were treated in the Chur Kantonsspital, most of them with severe injuries, and particularly those with fatal injuries (fig. 6/3), children requiring surgery (fig. 3/65) and collision cases (table 3/I).

One 'typical injury' was observed, namely depressed fractures in 84% of the operated cases (92% of children), some accompanied by brain contusion or brain hemorrhage.

A total of 66 cases of depressed fractures with or without hematoma/brain contusion were treated surgically (table 3/II). The age group up to 19 years clearly showed the highest accident rate, namely 45 cases (68%), most of these boys. Breakdown by sex shows a 4:1 ratio, i.e. 4 male patients to 1 female (in this discussion 50 men represent 76%).

The 'typical injuries' of the head that were observed bear out the importance of simple preventive measures in this sport [39, 41]. The severe

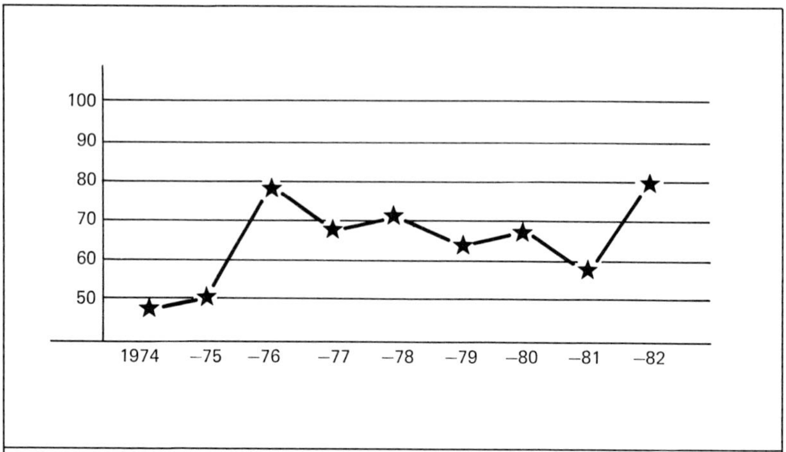

3/64

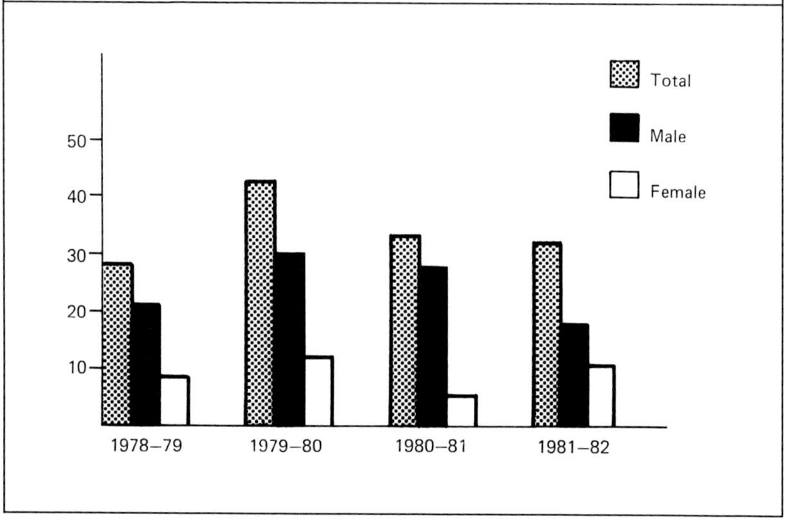

3/65

Fig. 3/64. Number of patients.
Fig. 3/65. Number of children.

injuries caused by collisions while skiing can be compared to injuries from collisions between cars on the road, in that slower skiers always suffer severe injuries caused by faster skiers (table 3/I).

The slightly injured (group b) were mostly young skiers and they were predominantly male, excessive speed and careless, uncontrolled skiing being the causes of the accidents.

Table 3/I. Cases of collisions

Patient No.	Severe injury (a) age/sex	→ collision ←	Minor injury (b) age/sex	Month
1	18/M		43/M	Feb.
2	65/F		14/M	Jan.
3	9/M		?	Mar.
4	16/M		18/M	Jan.
5	22/F*		17/M	Feb.
6	17/F		15/F	Feb.
7	51/M		17/M	Feb.
8	22/M*		?	Feb.
9	23/M		25/M	Jan.
10	16/M		34/M	Feb.
11	17/F		15/M	Feb.
12	11/F*		14/M	Jan.
13	8/F		11/M	Feb.
14	10/M		11/M	Feb.
15	17/M		?	Feb.
16	22/F		17/M	Feb.
17	36/F		22/M	Feb.
18	19/M		?	Mar.
19	47/M*		16/M	Mar.
20	28/F*		?	Mar.
21	47/M		27/M	Feb.

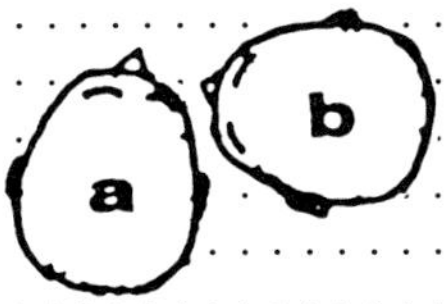

* Died.

Table 3/II. Age and sex of patients with depressed fracture

Age, years	Men	Women	Total
0–19	33	12	45
20–29	12	3	15
Over 30	5	1	6
Total	50	16	66

Table 3/III. Age and sex distribution of the fatal cases

Age, years	Sex		Total
	male	female	
9–19	5	1	6
20–25	3	1	5
26–40	3	1	4
41–50	1	1	2
Total	12	4	16

It is noteworthy that the largest number of accidents occurred in February (13 cases = 62%), this being caused by the 'traffic congestion' on the ski slopes during that month. It should be pointed out that, in collisions, one of the participants often suffers severe injuries whereas the other is only slightly injured or suffers no injuries at all.

All kinds of people take part in this popular winter sport, from children (the youngest was 3 years old) to the elderly (the oldest was 75 years), men and women, even including semi-invalids, and the growing number of skiers can cause an increasing number of accidents. In the course of 4 years (1978–1982) I have treated 138 children with head injuries (fig. 3/65).

28 children were treated surgically for depressed fractures [44]. Skiing for pleasure and for health has a much higher accident rate than has driving on the road, the figure being about 50,000 accidents during the 4-month winter season of 1967 in Switzerland. Many were tragic cases, as illustrated in figure 6/3. In comparison with other sports, the fatalities are particularly significant because children and young skiers were mainly involved (table 3/III).

Of 16 fatal cases, 10 were below 25 years of age, and 12 were male. 75%, i.e. the majority of the accidents, occurred during the month of February. The accidents were caused mainly by fast, uncontrolled skiing (no-one else involved). But slow and careful skiers also suffered fatal head injuries, mostly because of collision with a fast skier on an open slope (second person involved) (table 3/I).

The youngest victim was 9 and the oldest 47 years of age. It is remarkable that 7 deaths occurred in 1980 alone, 60% of them in the month of February. 11 of the 16 patients were injured in accidents involving only

Table 3/IV. Comparison with other authors' figures for the frequency of fatal skiing accidents

Injury	Haid (A) (1944–1954)	Pöschl (G) (1948–1957)	Oh (S) (1975–1982)
Head	9	13	16
General	5	4	/
Total	14	17	16

(A) = Austria; (G) = Germany; (S) = Switzerland.

themselves. In more than two thirds of the fatal skull injuries, no one else was involved in the accident (fall on open slope, deviation from normal slope, collision with obstacle, etc.). The causes of these accidents can be attributed to inadequate physical fitness and fast, careless skiing, as has also been observed by other authors [22, 25, 33, 50, 54]. Boys and young men are particularly prone to this type of accident (90% under 25 years old, the group at risk). One third of these fatal head injuries were not the victim's own fault, however. As a rule, these were suffered by slow and careful skiers run into by faster skiers on an open slope.

By comparison with neighboring countries, Switzerland has shown a higher rate of fatal cases (table 3/IV) in recent years.

4 Experimental Study

Of all the operations, more than 84% (children 92%) were performed for depressed fracture with or without brain damage or hemorrhage (fig. 4/1) [39, 43, 44, 46].

This is a typical type of head injury, which must be treated surgically in all cases and from which many consequences and complications may result [39, 41].

Thus, the experimental study was directed mainly at depressed skull fractures, namely fractures caused by the action of kinetic energy, the morphological effects on human skulls and model skulls being analyzed [24, 43, 45, 49]. The study concentrated mainly on the application of forces of direct local impact, which lead to depressed fractures.

Physical Conditions of Skiing

Skiing is a downward movement on an angled plane (fig. 4/2). The speed can be determined by the appropriate choice of angle and direction. Dividing the plane into 360°, with the 6 o'clock direction representing the line of greatest slope, the following possibilities should be considered: downhill skiing takes place within a 90° segment of the circle, and the choice of the angle determines the skiing direction – from a horizontal movement (3 o'clock) to the line of greatest slope (6 o'clock descent). The lowest speed is achieved by moving in the horizontal direction (for example cross-country skiing). The more the skiing direction approaches the line of greatest slope, the higher the speed becomes. In skiing regions, the degree of difficulty of a slope (fig. 4/3) is indicated by different color markings (degree of difficulty increasing from blue to red to black slopes). A skier reaches the highest speed when his descent approaches the line of greatest slope (downhill races).

The speed is also influenced by other factors, some of which can only partly be controlled by the skier, such as angle of slope (AS), snow condi-

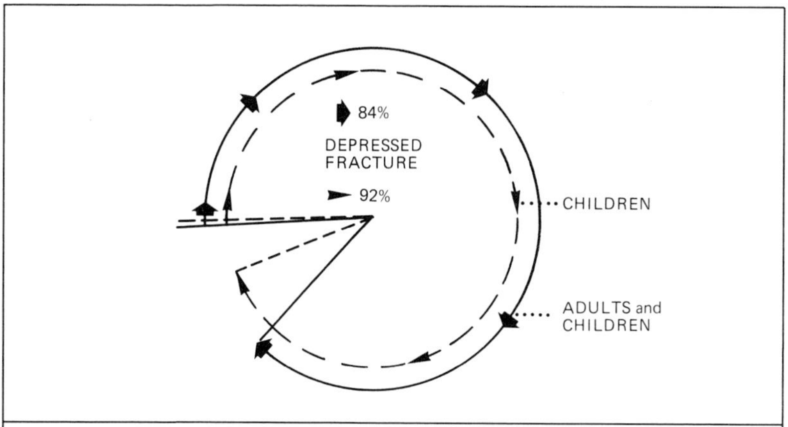

4/1

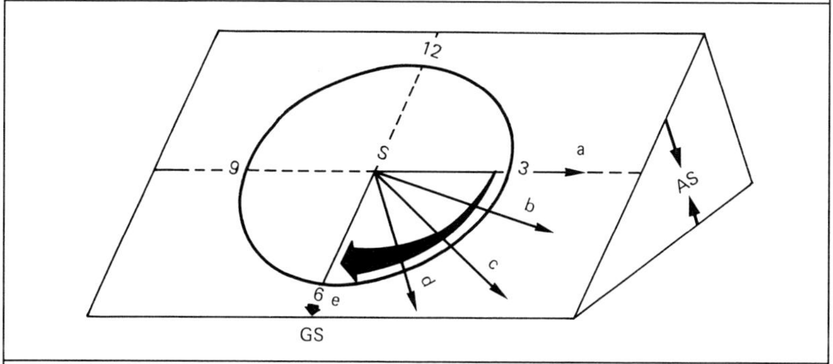

4/2

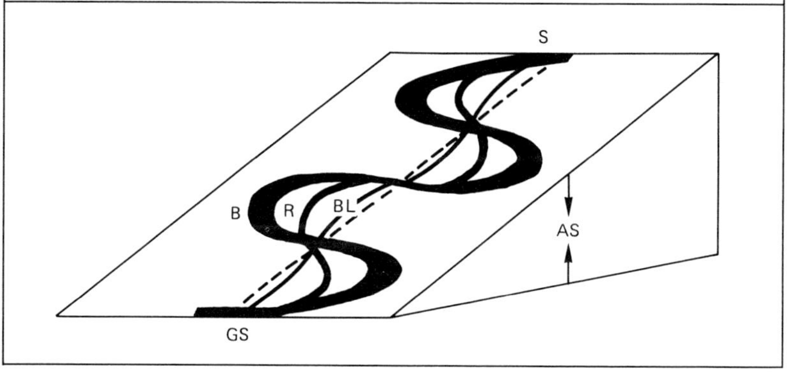

4/3

Fig. 4/1. Surgical cases (adults and children) showed more than 84% (children 92%) with depressed skull fractures.

Fig. 4/2. The closer the skiing direction approaches the line of greatest slope the higher the downhill speed becomes. AS = Angle of slope; S = starting point; GS = line of greatest slope.

Fig. 4/3. Ski slope markings. BL = Black slope; B = blue slope; R = red slope.

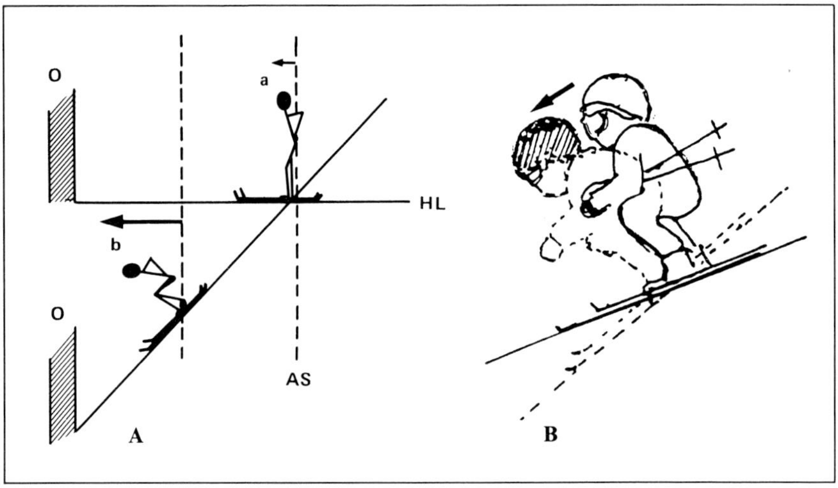

Fig. 4/4. A Head position in the crouched position of a high-speed skier (b), in comparison with a cross-country skier (a). a = Cross-country skiing; b = downhill skiing; HL = horizontal line; O = obstacle. **B** High-speed skier assumes head-forward position automatically.

tions (ice, powder or slush), preparation of slope, and skier's equipment and body weight.

When skiing at high speed on a steep slope, the head of the skier (in contrast to slow-speed skiing) is always in the most forward position by virtue of the weight distribution and for aerodynamic reasons (fig. 4/4A, B).

High-speed skiing in this crouched position is especially dangerous, because when colliding with an obstacle, the head, being the first part of the body to strike, absorbs the full kinetic energy and thus severe head injury is the main and often the only result.

Skull Injuries from the Application of Force

Different kinds of skull fractures (fig. 4/5, C) occur depending on the impact energy and impulse (fig. 4/5, A), which themselves are dependent on the part of the head hit (fig. 4/5, B).

The type and extent of these injuries also vary depending on the point of impact on the head (fig. 4/6) [59], and on the characteristics of the latter,

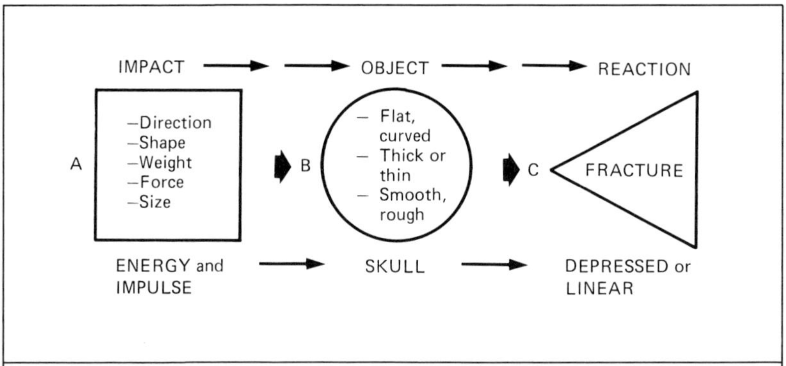

4/5

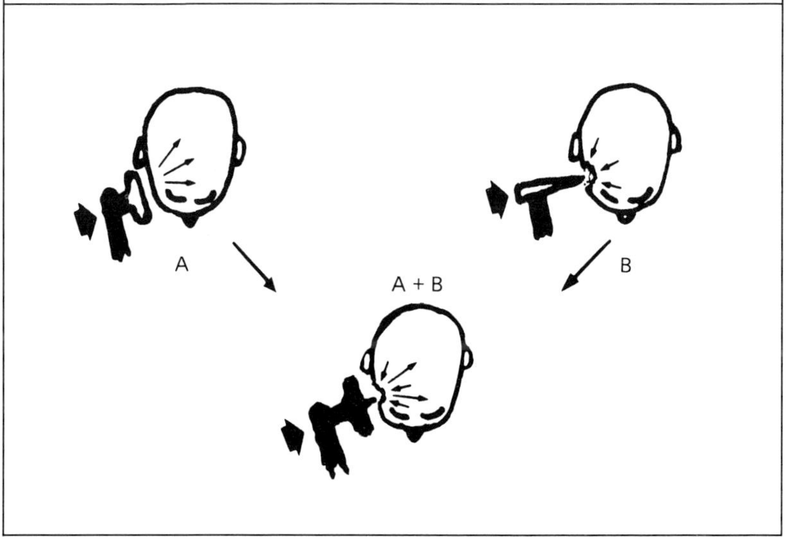

4/6

Fig. 4/5. Circumstances leading to fracture.
Fig. 4/6. The impact of different shapes causes different injury patterns.

as well as on the nature of the objects' injuries affecting either the skull alone (fig. 4/6, B), the brain (fig. 4/6, A) or skull and brain together (fig. 4/6, A + B) will result [4, 19]. Based on the objects' impact, there are therefore three categories of head injuries, i.e. large or small surface area, as well as a mixed type.

Application of force over a large area (fig. 4/7) leads almost exclusively to brain contusion, with or without a linear fracture (fig. 4/8) [49].

4/7
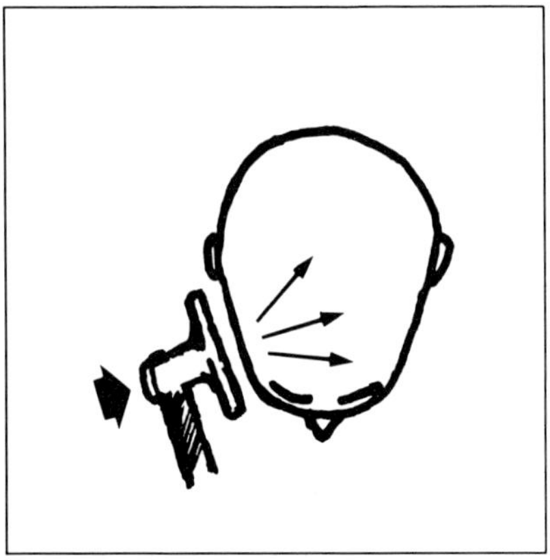

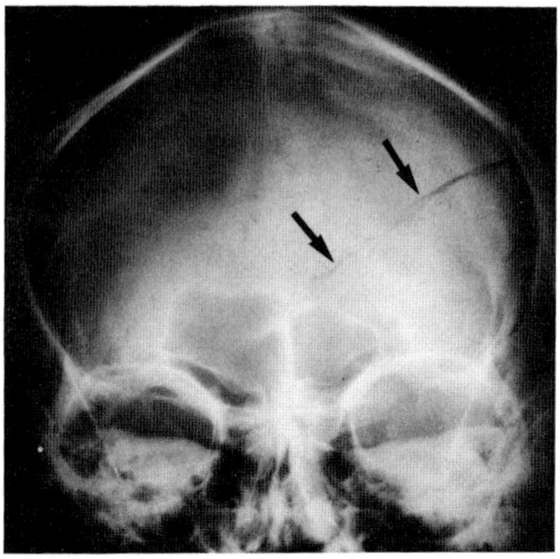
4/8

4/9
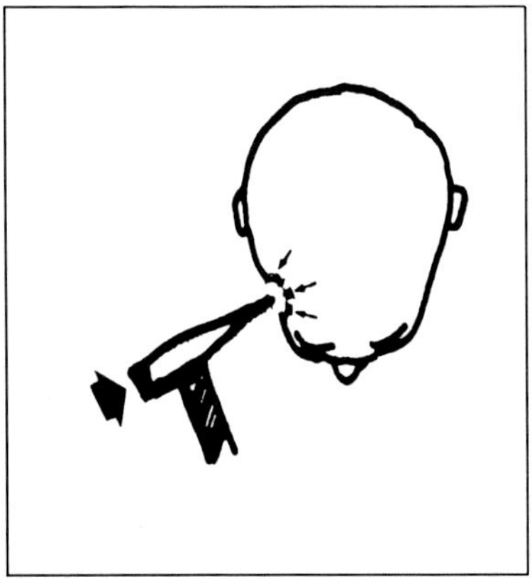

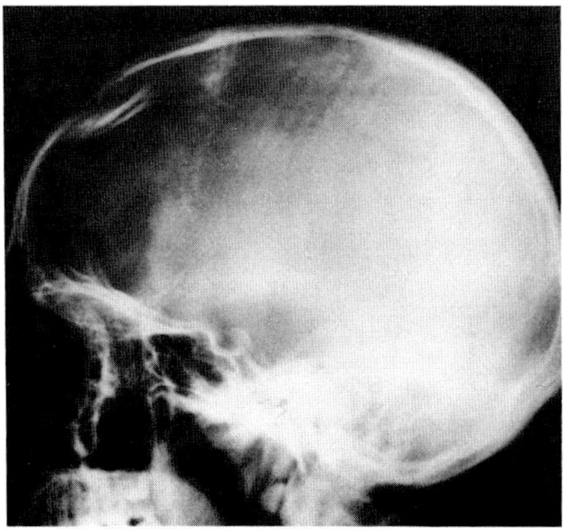
4/10

Fig. 4/7. Application of force over a large area causes mainly brain contusion with or without linear fracture.

Fig. 4/8. A fall on the hard ski slope at high speed leading to a linear fracture with brain contusion.

Fig. 4/9. Application of force over small area causes depressed fracture.

Fig. 4/10. Depressed fracture, with or without brain damage (struck by ski-lift T-bar).

Impact of force over a small area (fig. 4/9) usually results in depressed fractures, with or without brain damage (fig. 4/10), and these occur particularly often during skiing and require surgical reconstruction.

Collision with a boulder having flat and pointed areas (fig. 4/11) results in a mixed skull fracture, such as a compound, comminuted, depressed

4/11

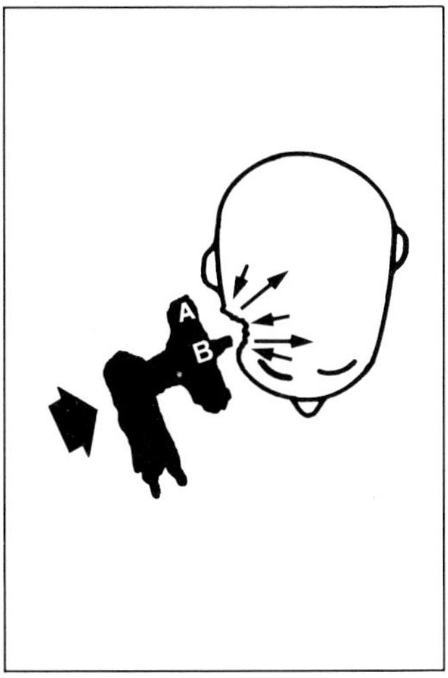

4/12

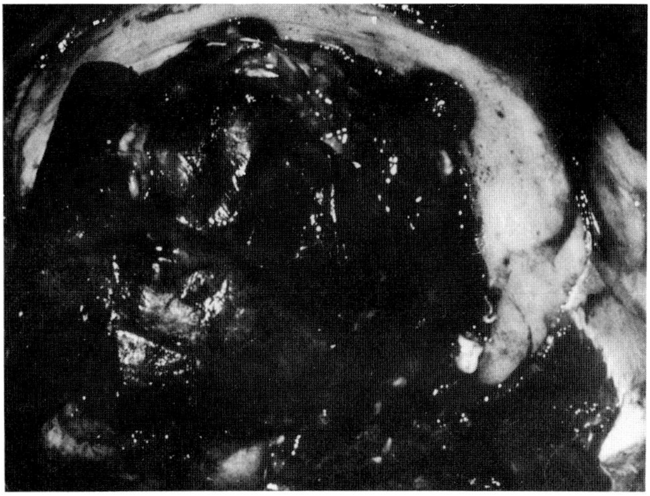

Fig. 4/11. Application of force over both a small (B) and a large area (A).
Fig. 4/12. Severe craniocerebral injury (mixed type).

skull fracture (fig. 4/12). As figure 4/11 illustrates, a mixed fracture is produced, as can be seen with case 20 (fig. 3/34), a so-called compound, comminuted, depressed skull fracture with severe brain contusion (fig. 4/12). The first result is penetration damage, namely the depressed fracture, and then decerebration injury, i.e. brain contusion.

This can be seen with case 20, a 40-year-old man, who hit his head directly against a boulder, and suffered an extensive compound, comminuted, depressed fracture with severe brain contusion.

Experimental Study of Depressed Skull Fracture

Experimental Procedure

A partitioned skull was fixed tightly with glue and was placed between two pieces of soft material which supported its weight yet permitted virtually free movement of the skull for the dynamic test.

In a free fall experiment, a cylindrical steel body with a spherical impact surface of radius of curvature 14 mm was allowed to fall onto the skull. Additional weights could be screwed onto the steel body, and an

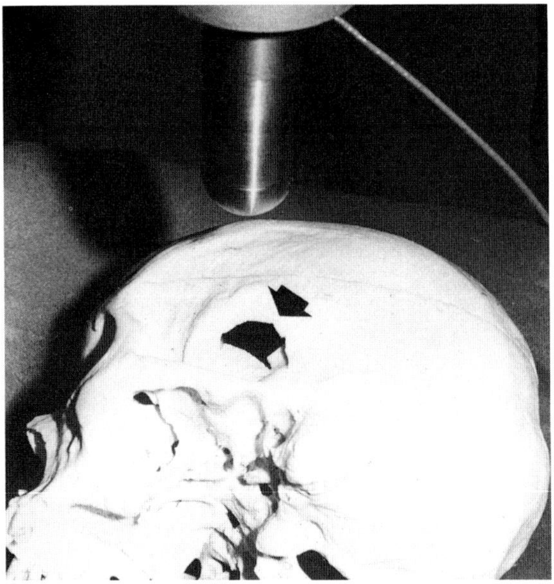

Fig. 4/13. Impactor, with acceleration indicator.

acceleration indicator was mounted in it, which showed a current proportionate to the acceleration (fig. 4/13).

By means of a current amplifier, this was transformed into a voltage signal which was stored digitally in a transient recorder. Slowed down 1,000-fold, the acceleration time curve was recorded on a chart recorder (fig. 4/14).

The tested part of the skull was covered during the test with moistened leather about 4 mm thick in order to simulate the damping effect of the scalp. This procedure also improved the measurement of acceleration. With undampened impacts, self-oscillation of the measuring system sometimes occurs.

Sites of Impact and Results

Most tests were carried out on the temporal areas (right and left), but other regions were also tested (frontal region). After macroscopic inspection, the fractures were described and recorded photographically. Nine

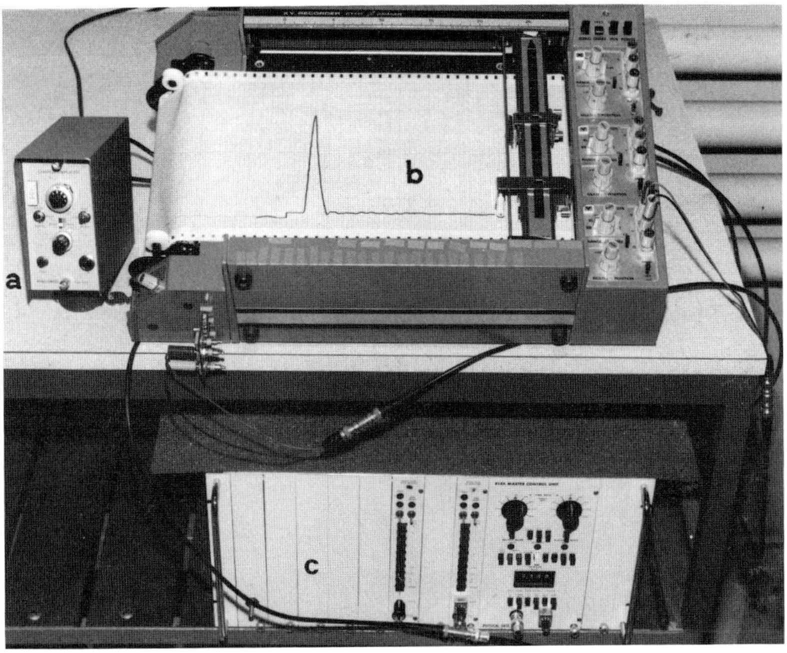

Fig. 4/14. Measuring apparatus. a = Current-amplifier; b = chart-recorder; c = transient recorder.

skulls were tested, with a total of 38 dynamic tests, of which 23 were performed in the temporal and 15 in the frontal area (table 4/I).

For comparison, the tests were also conducted in the frontal regions (fig. 4/15). The measured forces were much higher than those in the temporal region. Often, a fracture could not be produced even at greatly increased impact energies. The reason is certainly that the skull bones in the frontal region are more than 3 times as thick (table 4/II).

After the tests the skulls were broken and their thicknesses measured (table 4/II).

The results of the impact experiments in the temporal and frontal regions are listed in table 4/I. In some individual tests the acceleration lies outside the fixed measuring limits (test 2, etc.). During other tests, the acceleration could not be determined exactly because of self-oscillation of the system (e.g. tests 11 and 12). Tests for which the acceleration was not

Table 4/I. Results of the impact experiments in the temporal and frontal areas

Test No. 1	Fall height, m 2	Fall weight, kg 3	Energy J 4	Speed km/h 5	Accelera-tion, *g* 6	Force kN 7	Skull No. 8	Fracture 9
Temporal								
2	2.7	1.39	37	26.2	> 100	> 1.4	2	+++
3	2.7	1.39	37	26.2	> 100	> 1.4	2	+++
4	1.0	1.39	14	15.9	> 100	> 1.4	2	++
11	0.7	1.39	10	13.3	~ 130	~ 1.8	1	0
12	1.0	1.39	14	15.9	~ 110	~ 1.5	1	+
13	0.8	1.39	11	14.3	120	1.6	1	++
14	0.9	1.39	12	15.1	0	0.0	1	+
15	0.9	1.39	12	15.1	~ 150	~ 2.0	1	+
24	0.8	1.39	11	14.3	65	0.9	3	0
25	1.0	1.39	14	15.9	0	0.0	3	+++
26	0.8	1.39	11	14.4	55	0.7	3	+++
27	1.0	1.39	14	15.9	80	1.1	3	++
28	0.8	1.39	11	14.3	80	1.1	4	++
29	0.8	1.39	11	14.3	85	1.2	4	++
33	0.8	1.39	11	14.3	~ 120	~ 1.6	5	++
34	0.8	1.39	11	14.3	90	1.2	5	++
38	0.8	1.39	11	14.3	75	1.0	6	+++
39	0.7	1.39	10	13.3	70	1.0	6	++
40	0.8	1.39	11	14.3	130	1.8	7	+
41	0.8	1.39	11	14.3	105	1.4	7	0
42	0.8	1.39	11	14.3	90	1.2	7	+
43	1.0	1.39	14	15.9	125	1.7	8	++
44	1.0	1.39	14	15.9	100	1.4	8	++
Frontal								
5	1.0	1.39	14	15.9	~ 200	~ 2.7	2	0
6	1.5	1.39	20	19.5	200	2.7	2	+
16	1.5	1.39	20	19.5	~ 320	~ 4.4	1	+
17	1.5	1.39	20	19.5	~ 310	~ 4.2	1	+
18	2.0	1.39	27	22.5	320	4.4	1	+
22	1.0	1.39	14	15.9	85	1.2	3	0
23	1.0	1.39	14	15.9	180	2.5	3	0
30	1.5	1.39	20	19.5	210	2.9	4	0
31	2.0	1.39	27	22.5	175	2.4	4	0
32	2.7	1.39	37	26.2	230	3.1	4	0
35	2.7	1.39	37	26.2	300	4.1	5	0
36	2.7	1.89	50	26.2	~ 210	~ 3.9	5	0
37	2.7	1.89	50	26.2	130	2.4	5	0
46	2.7	2.39	63	26.2	130	3.0	9	0
47	2.7	2.39	63	26.2	180	4.2	9	0

Column 9: 0 = no fracture; + = slight fracture; ++ = depressed fracture; +++ = total depressed fracture.

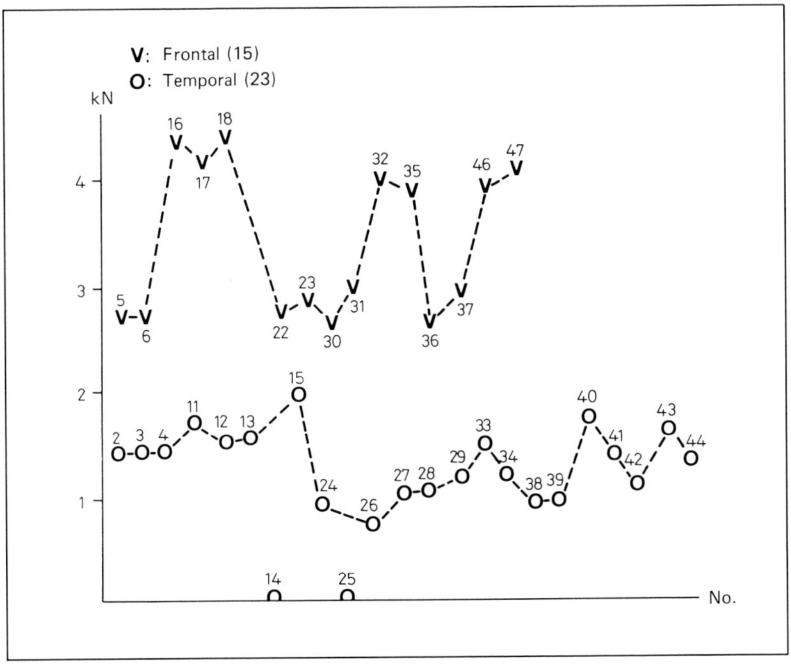

Fig. 4/15. Comparison of forces in the temporal and frontal regions (test No. corresponds to column 1 in table 4/I).

Table 4/II. Thickness of skulls (mm)

Skull No.	Age/sex	Location			
		frontal		temporal	
		right	left	right	left
1	unknown	10	9.5	2	2
2	ca. 40/F	9	9	2	1.5
3	ca. 50/M	8	7	2	1.5
4	ca. 50/M	9.5	9.5	2	2
5	unknown	9	9	1.5	2
6	ca. 55/M	8	8	1.5	1.5
7	unknown	7	7	1.5	2
8	ca. 70/M	8	8.5	2	2
9	ca. 25/M	7.5	7.5	2	2

4/16 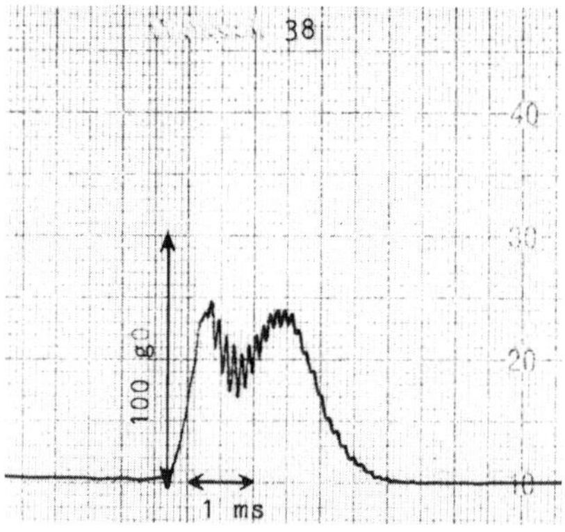

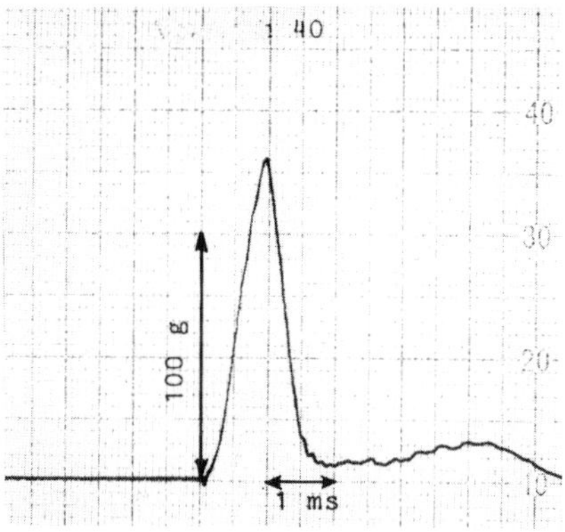 4/17

Fig. 4/16. Acceleration-time curve of a total depressed fracture (test 38).
Fig. 4/17. Acceleration-time curve of a slightly depressed fracture (test 40).

measured are identified in columns 6 and 7 by 'O' (tests 14 and 25). The acceleration-time curves from tests 38 and 40 are shown in figures 4/16 and 4/17. Test 38 resulted in a totally depressed fracture (fig. 4/18), whereas test 40 yielded only a slight depression (fig. 4/19).

Generally, it was observed that there was a tendency in cases of fracture for the measured acceleration (forces) to be smaller than when the skull remained intact. Of course this is true only for comparable energies. The reason for this is that, in the case of a fracture, the falling body is slowed down less than in the case of nonfracture.

In an accident, the energy of impact increases with the square of the speed.

Due to the ever-increasing speeds, this effect operates in various types of sport and in traffic accidents. The application of a low force to the skull may lead to depressed fractures, which is often the case in serious skiing accidents.

This study indicated a tolerance threshold of about 1–2 kN for a depressed fracture in the temporal area. The energy that leads to fractures in this area can be compared to a speed at about 16 km/h or to a fall from a height of 1 m.

For a fracture in the frontal region, application of a much greater force is required because the bones of the skull are more than three times as thick here. Slightly depressed fractures were found in this region in tests with 2.5–4.5 kN (table 4/I, fig. 4/15).

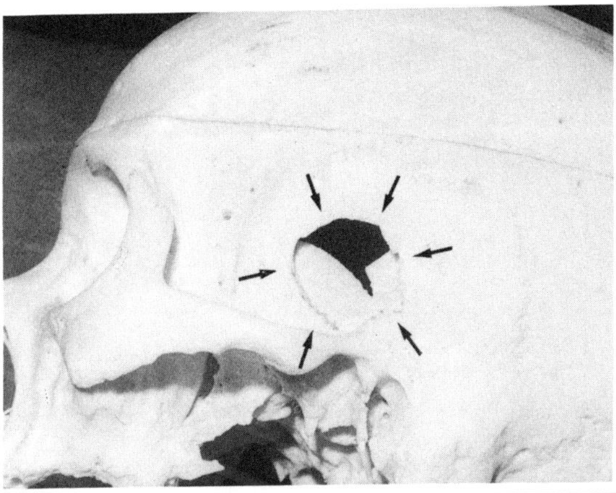

4/18

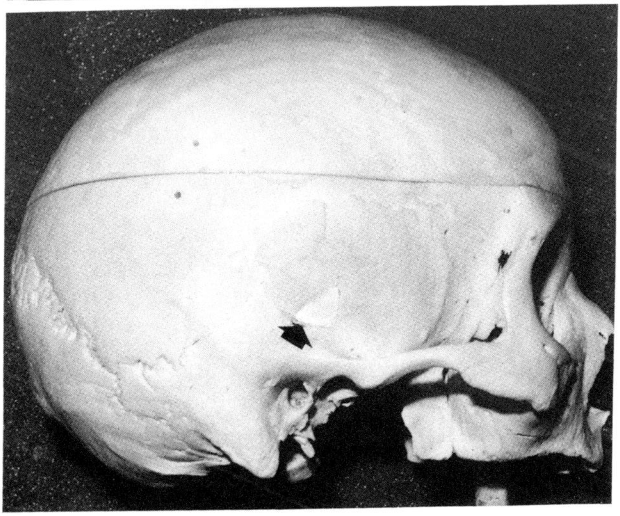

4/19

Fig. 4/18. Completely depressed fracture (test 38).
Fig. 4/19. Slightly depressed fracture (test 40).

The Reaction to the Energy of Impact

The severity and extent of injuries to the human cranium depend on the area over which the force is applied. The configuration of the human skull is characterised by two types of differently shaped surfaces (fig. 4/20). In the frontal and occipital regions the vault is curved and thick. The temporoparietal region has a flat surface and is thin [30].

4/20 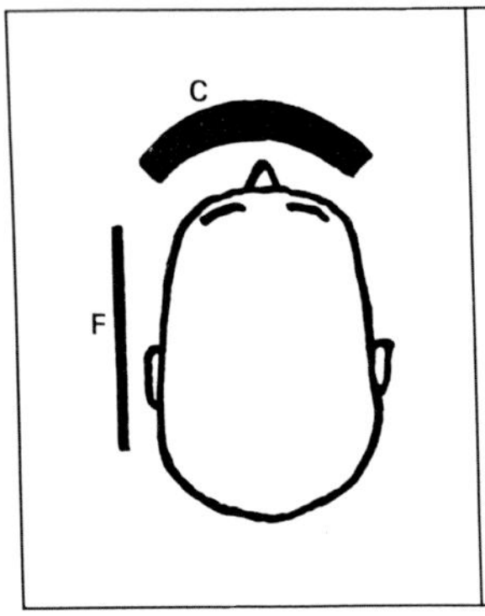

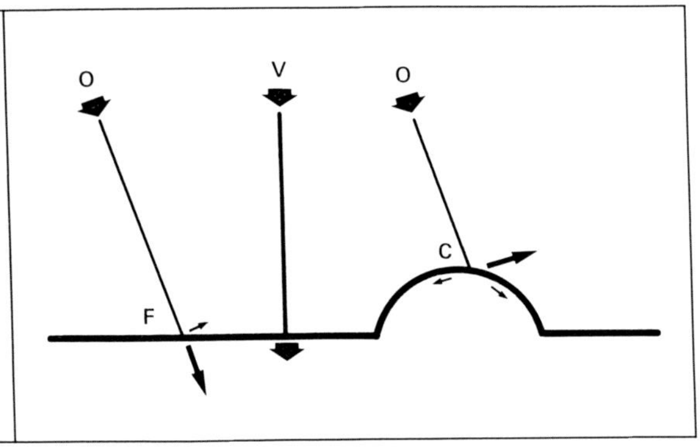 4/21

Fig. 4/20. The two different skull contours and thicknesses. C = Curved and thick; F = flat and thin.

Fig. 4/21. Reaction to the application of force. For details see text.

Important brain functions (motor and speech, etc.) and important vessels (middle cerebral vessels) are located in the weaker region. For these histo-anatomical and functional reasons, injuries to the lateral area of the head occur more easily and often during skiing, and they may then result in particularly serious damage and complications. Many fewer craniocerebral injuries occur from physical reactions in the thick, curved frontal and occipital regions, because most of the impact force is deflected (fig. 4/21, C).

In experimental studies, a bolt of low surface area and weight of 3 kg was allowed to fall from a height of 80–100 cm onto the temporoparietal region of various human crania in different positions and, depending on the angle of impact (or angle of the target), quite different injury patterns were found.

Virtually all of a vertical force (fig. 4/22) is absorbed by the skull and, in particular, an object of small surface area hitting the flat temporoparietal region will cause a depressed fracture (fig. 4/23).

In contrast, objects impinging at an angle (fig. 4/21, O) are much less dangerous, because most of the force applied to the skull is deflected and thus only a part of the kinetic energy is absorbed by the bone of the skull (fig. 4/24). I have observed this and documented it by cinematography in experimental studies on the human skull (fig. 4/24, 4/25) [43].

Compared with a vertical force (fig. 4/21, V), the effect of application of an oblique force is less on a flat surface (fig. 4/21, F), because much more of the kinetic energy is deflected and therefore less force is absorbed by the

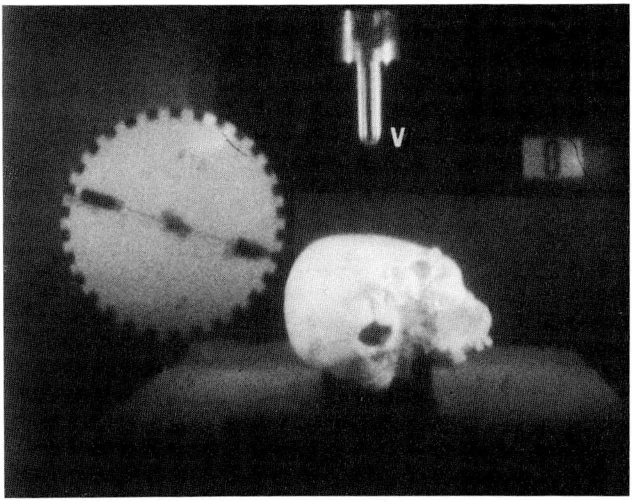

Fig. 4/22. Impact of the falling body with a vertical force (V) results in a depressed fracture.

surface. For the same reason, a blow on a curved surface (fig. 4/21, C) will have less serious consequences than the same blow on a flat surface.

I have found that in skiers the temporoparietal area is particularly prone to serious injury for the following reasons: (1) On a curved surface, the impinging object will be deflected more than on a flat surface. Thus, in the case of the human skull, the effect of the oblique force component is strongly influenced by the nature of the surface of the cranium (fig. 4/20, F). Against the smooth curved surface of the thick frontal bone a blow will have practically no effect (fig. 4/20, C), for most of the energy is deflected and the bone withstands the remaining energy (fig. 4/26, C). Conversely, the rough, flat and comparatively thin bone of the parietotemporal region (fig. 4/22) will only deflect a small percentage of the kinetic energy of impact and the blow will result in a fracture (fig. 4/23). (2) Moreover, a curved structure is capable of absorbing a large force by diverting it along the curve to its base (fig. 4/26, C) – a static advantage of the arch known to architects since ancient times. On the other hand, a flat surface conducts the energy of impact directly to the underlying tissues (fig. 4/26, F), which means cranio-cerebral damage in the parietotemporal region, because of the rather flat anatomical configuration.

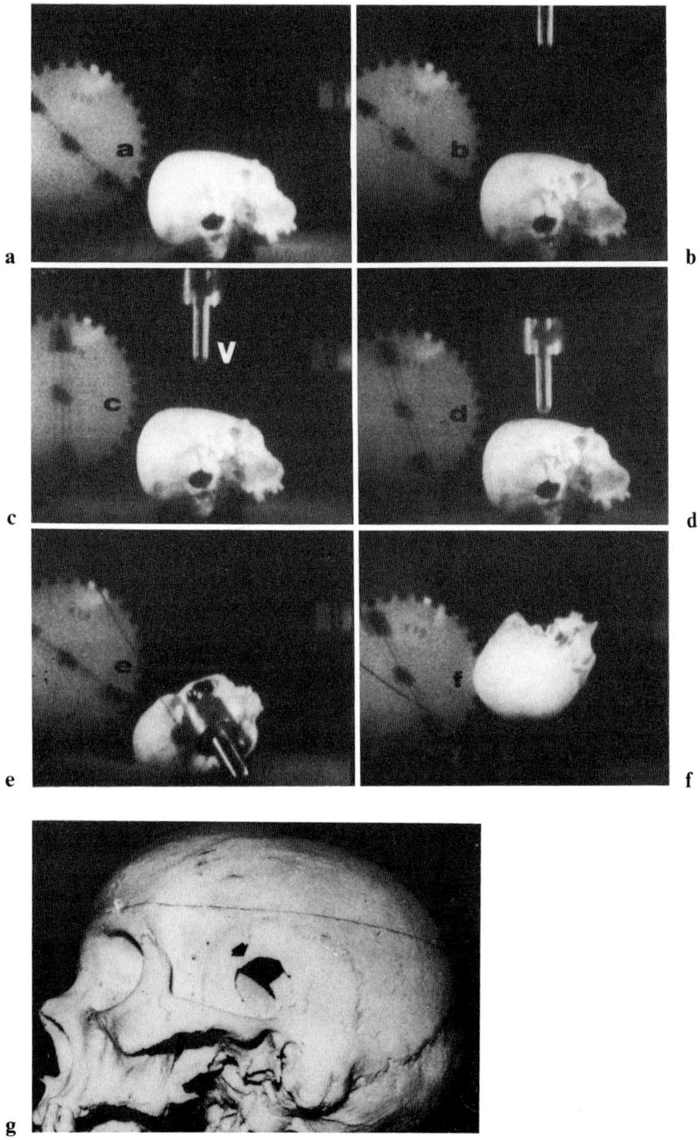

Fig. 4/23. Bolt dropping vertically onto the temporoparietal region (**a**–**f**) results in a depressed fracture (**g**).

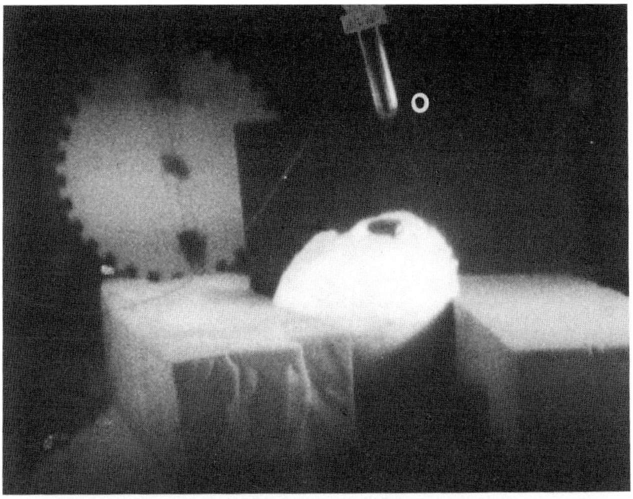

4/24

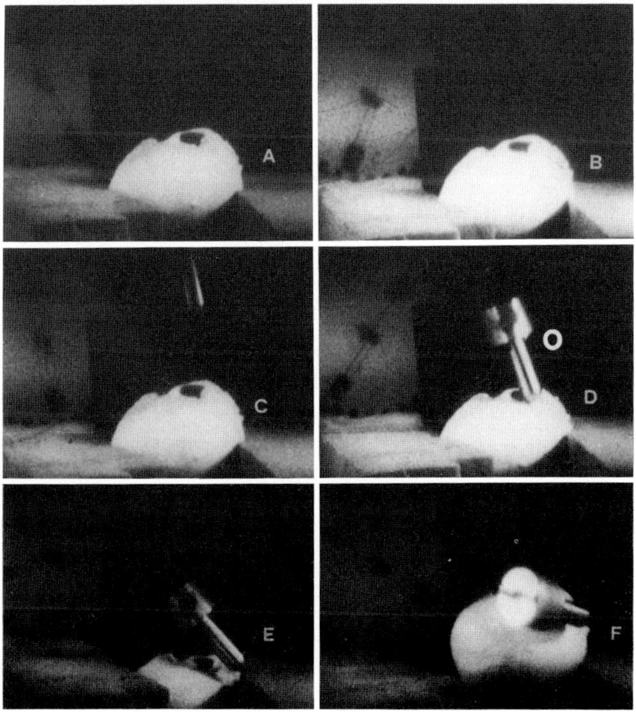

4/25

Fig. 4/24. Oblique energy (O) impact of the falling body without fracture.

Fig. 4/25. Bolt hitting the same skull region at an angle does not cause a depressed skull fracture.

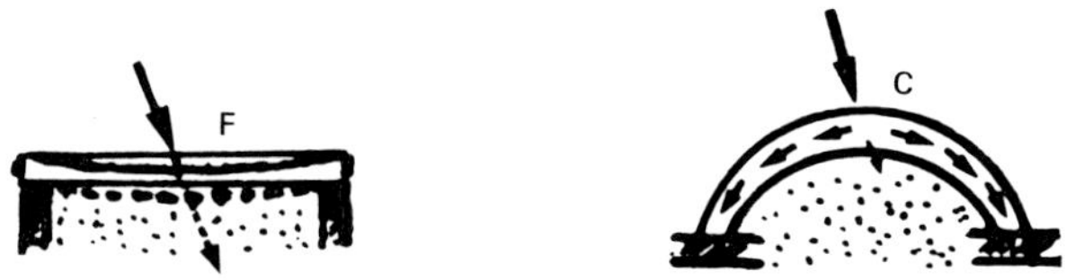

Fig. 4/26. Energy impinging on a flat surface has a penetrating effect (F). Energy impinging on a curved and smooth surface is deflected or conducted to its base (C).

Clinical and Experimental Study of the Morphology of the Depressed Fracture

Clinical Study

Between 1974 and 1982 (8 years) I treated 109 patients with depressed fractures surgically (fig. 4/27).

A large proportion of these depressed fractures derived from skiing accidents (66 patients, 61%). The rest were from traffic accidents, falls or thrown stones, etc. Often, depressed fractures are caused by collision with a variety of obstacles, such as: accidents caused by contact with a ski-tip (fig. 4/28, 4/29); thrown stone (fig. 4/30); collision with a boulder (fig. 4/31).

A CT scan shows the morphology of a depressed fracture clearly, with larger fracture of the inner table than of the outer (fig. 4/29). A depressed fracture with or without brain contusion caused by a thrown stone can be seen in figure 4/30. Clinically, the morphological structure is as in figure

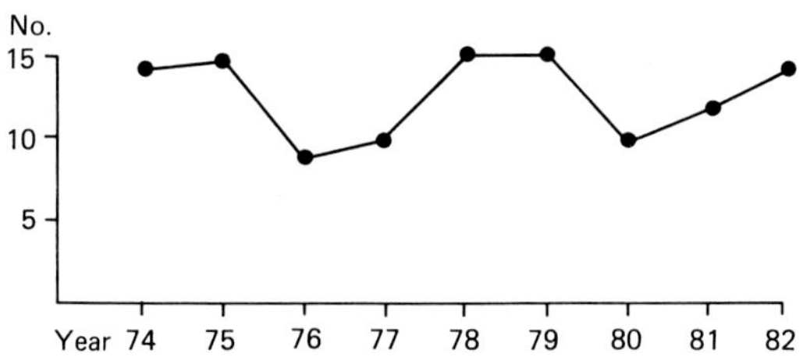

Fig. 4/27. Number of patients with depressed fractures treated surgically.

4/28

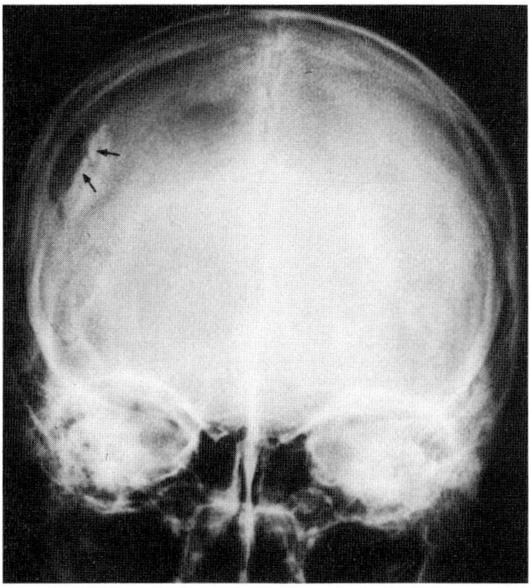

4/29

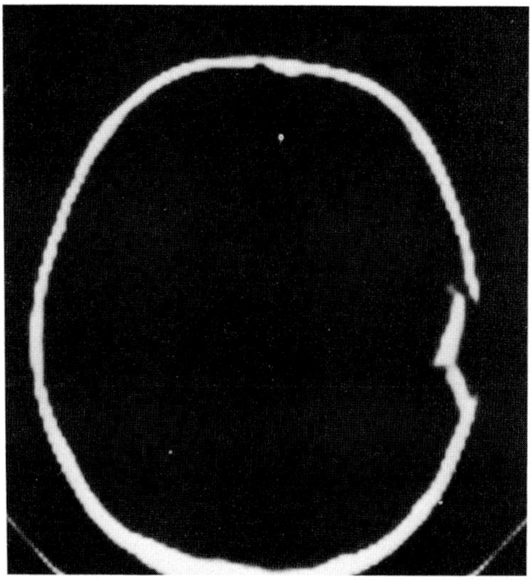

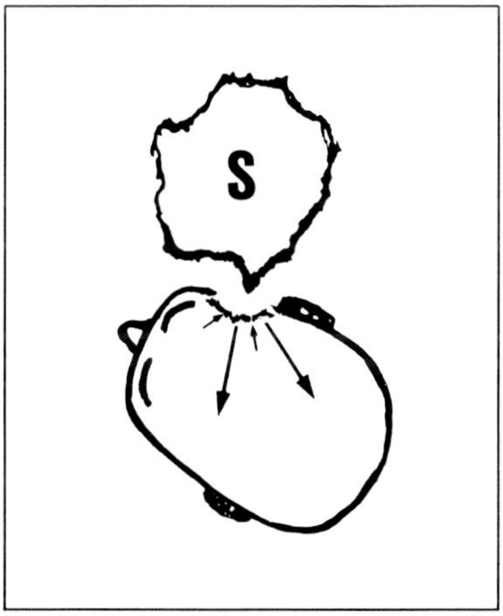

4/30

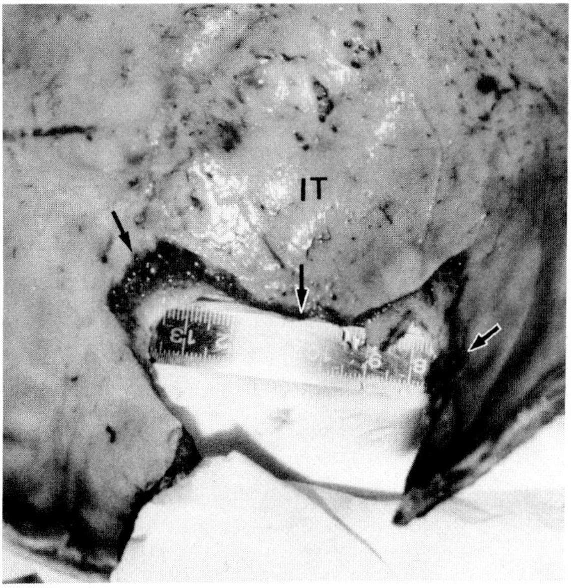

4/31

Fig. 4/28. Depressed fracture in right parietal region caused by ski-tip.

Fig. 4/29. CT scan showing the morphological structure of the depressed fracture.

Fig. 4/30. Thrown stone. S = Stone.

Fig. 4/31. A depressed fracture, the inner table having a larger fracture than the outer table. IT = Inner table.

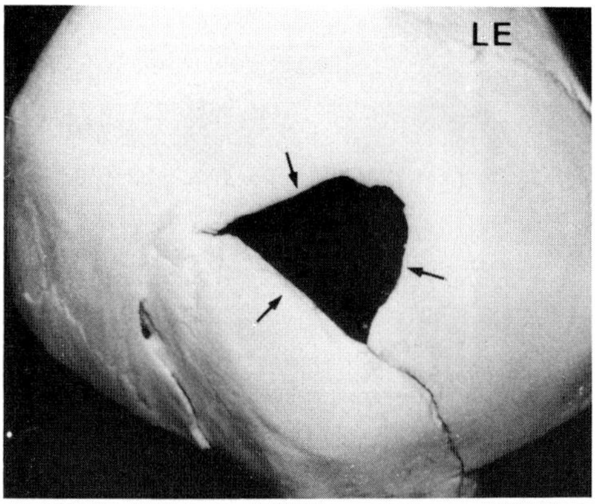

4/32A

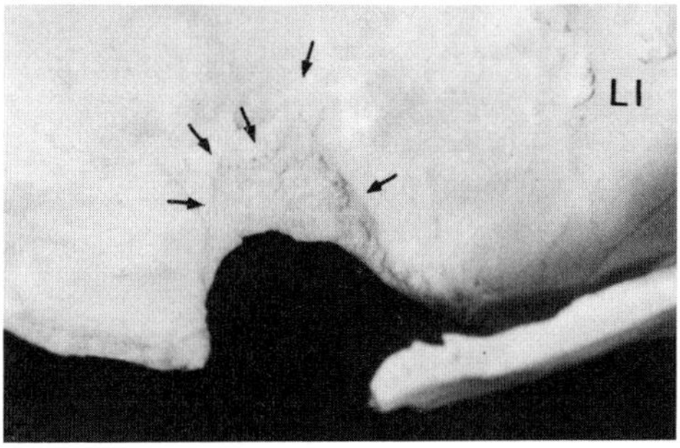

4/32B

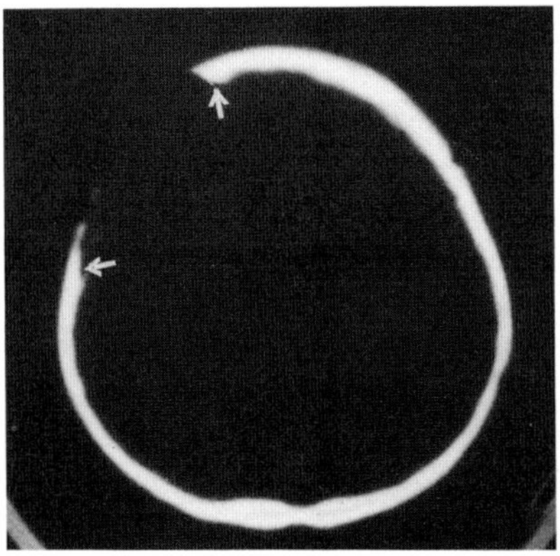

Fig. 4/32. Autopsy findings. Smaller fracture of the outer table (**A**). Larger fracture of the inner table (**B**).

Fig. 4/33. CT scan revealed the typical morphological form of the depressed fracture.

4/23, that is a larger fracture of the inner table than of the outer layer (fig. 4/31).

During the surgical treatment of depressed fractures, the morphological characteristic is that the fracture of the lamina interna is always larger than that of the lamina externa (fig. 4/32, 4/33) [45].

Experimental Morphological Study

Human Skulls

Clinically and experimentally, the same morphological patterns were always observed, that is, the fracture of the lamina interna is always larger than that of the outer table to an extent depending on the direction of impact (fig. 4/34).

Table 4/III. Depressed fracture results: method 1 (impact force: LE–LI)

Patient No.	Test No.	Skull No.	Fracture	Region
1	4	2	++	F
2	6	1	+	F
3	16	1	+	F
4	29	4	+	F
5	2	2	+++	T
6	3	2	+++	T
7	11	1	+	T
8	13	1	++	T
9	25	3	+++	T
10	26	3	+++	T
11	27	4	++	T
12	28	4	++	T
13	33	5	++	T
14	34	5	++	T
15	38	6	+++	T
16	39	6	++	T
17	40	7	+	T
18	42	7	+	T
19	43	8	++	T
20	44	9	++	T
21	14	1	+	P
22	15	1	+	P
23	53	10	+++	P
24	54	10	++	P

F = Frontal; T = temporal; P = parietal; LE = lamina externa; LI = lamina interna; + = slight fracture; ++ = depressed fracture; +++ = total depressed fracture.

The present morphological study was based on previously used skulls, in which 34 depressed fractures had been produced. 24 of these fractures derived from impact forces directed from the outer table towards the inner table, which is the only type occurring in clinical situations (table 4/III).

On the other hand, I made attempts to cause a depressed fracture from the inner table to the outer table (LI→LE). 10 depressed fractures were

Table 4/IV. Depressed fracture results: method 2 (impact force: LI-LE)

Patient No.	Test No.	Skull No.	Fracture	Region
1	55	6	++	P
2	56	6	+++	P
3	57	5	+++	O
4	59	4	+++	O
5	60	10	+++	P
6	61	4	++	P
7	62	3	++	P
8	65	7	++	P
9	66	2	+++	O
10	67	1	+++	O

P = Parietal; O = occipital; LI = lamina interna; LE = lamina externa.

produced (table 4/IV). It was now found that the fracture of the inner table was always smaller than that of the outer table (fig. 4/35). Of course, these types of depressed fractures would not be seen clinically.

Model Materials

Basically, there are three types of materials, namely soft (S), hard (H) and combination (C). In the following experimental study I used plasticine as the soft material and Palacos® (polymethyl methacrylate) as the hard material. From each material I made up various types and sizes of plates (fig. 4/36) and I studied the experimental procedure necessary to produce depressed fractures.

In experiments, I found the following: plasticine (S) gives neither a linear nor a depressed fracture. It spreads in all directions (fig. 4/37, 1). Palacos plates (H) show only linear fractures, even when a pointed impactor was used (fig. 4/36, 4/37, 2).

Fig. 4/34. **A** Larger fracture of the inner table (LI). **B** X-ray image shows larger fracture of the inner table (LI) and smaller fracture of the outer table (LE). **C** CT reveals larger fracture of the 'LI' than 'LE'.

Fig. 4/35. **A** Smaller fracture of inner table than of outer table. **B** CT scan shows clearly the larger fracture of the outer table than of the inner table. **C** The fragment from the fracture.

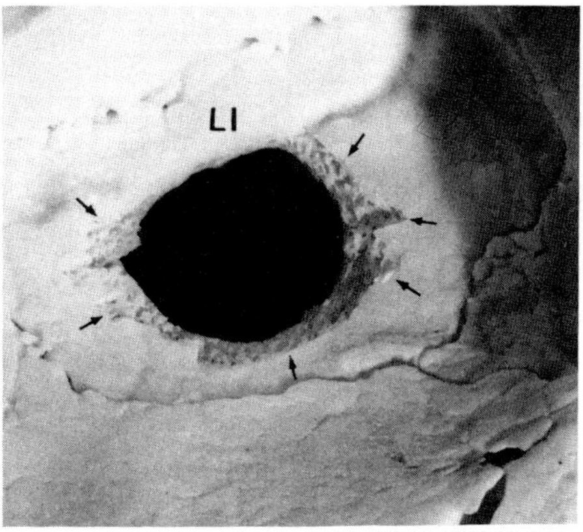

4/34A

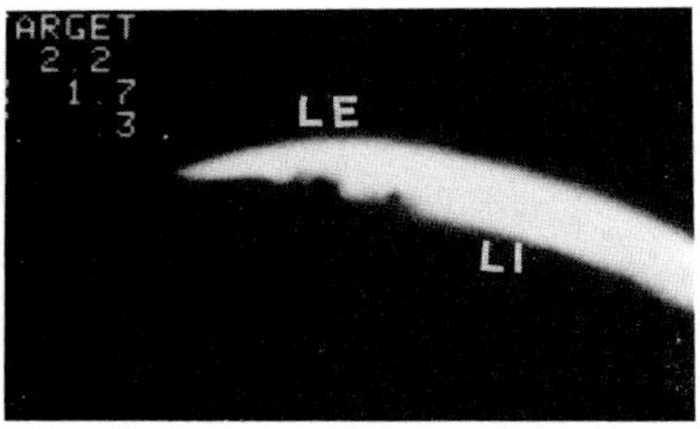

4/34C

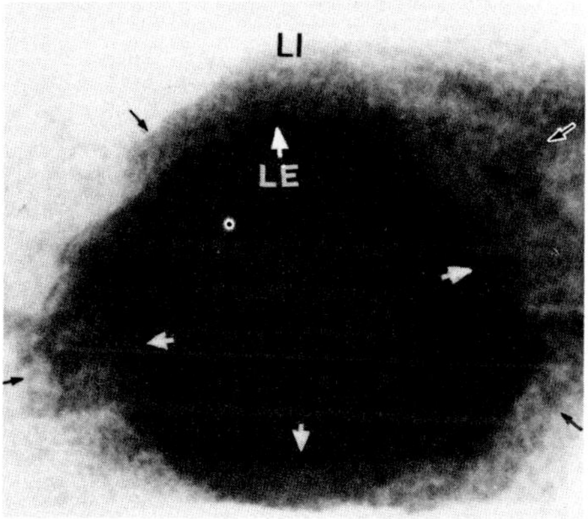

4/34B

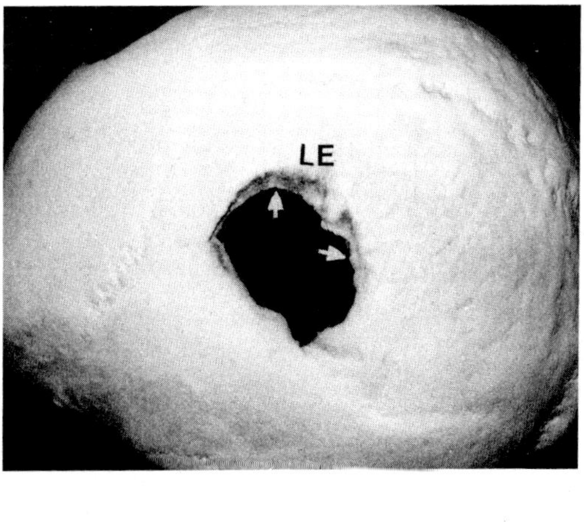

4/35A

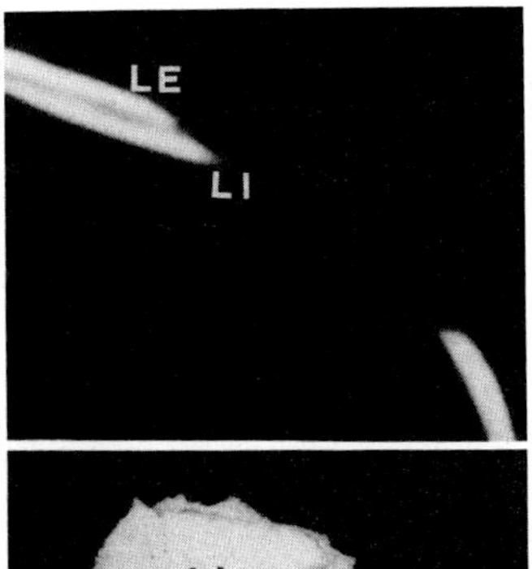

4/35B

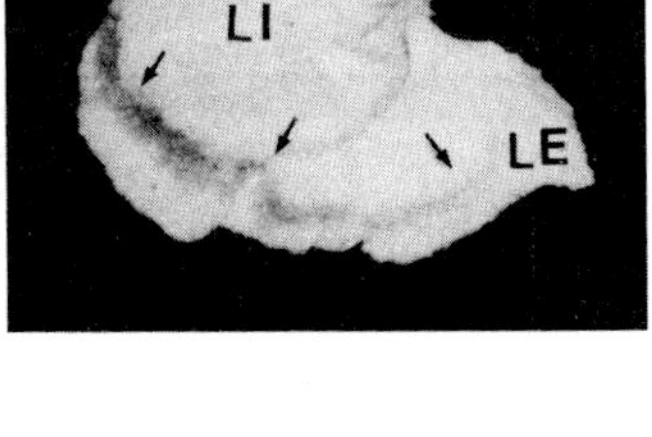

4/35C

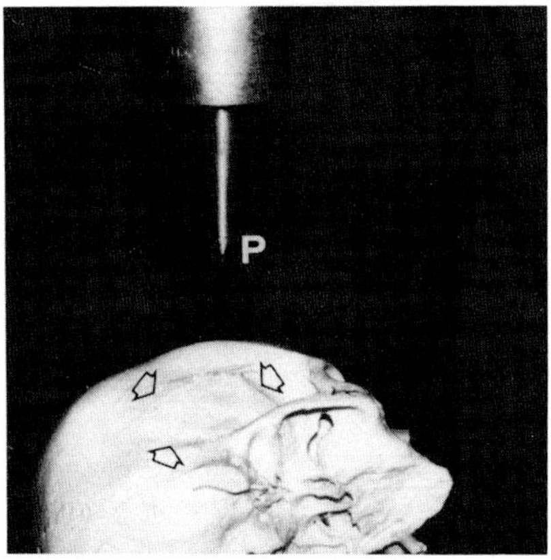

4/36A

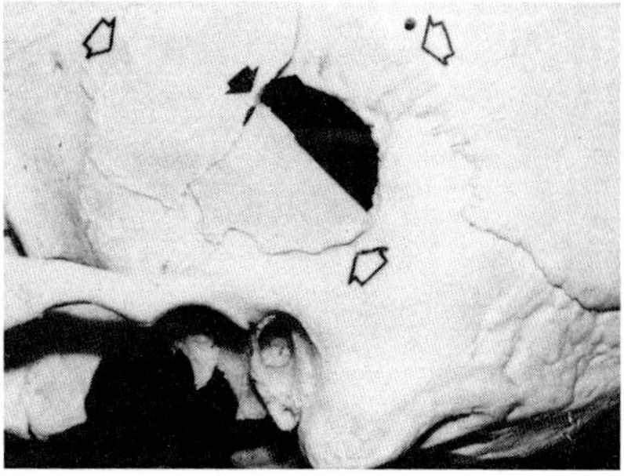

4.

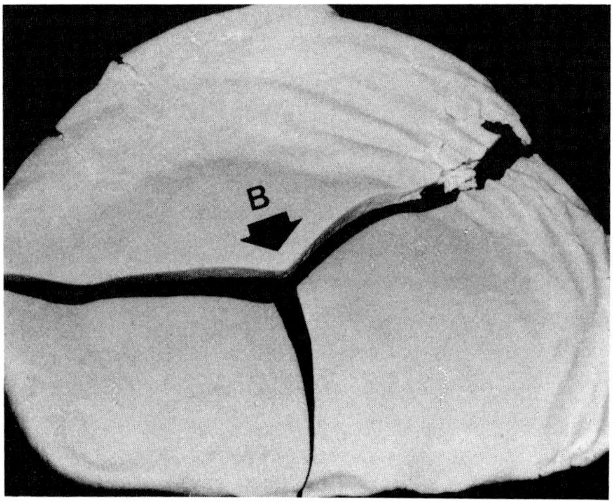

4/36C

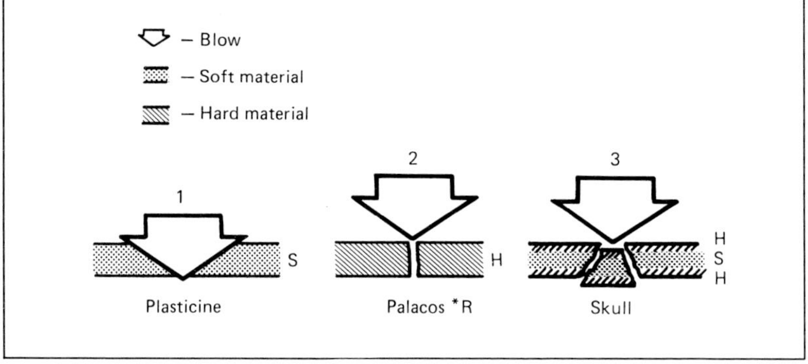

4/37

4/38

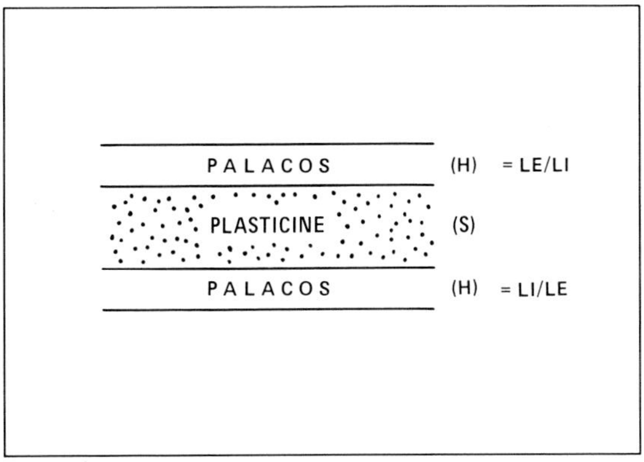

4/39

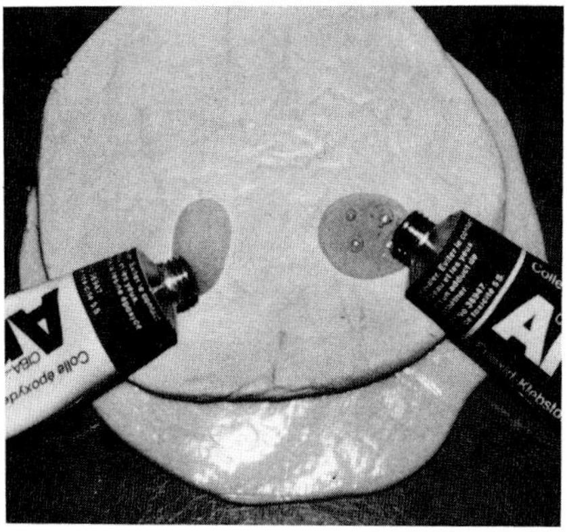

Fig. 4/38. Illustration of 'HSH' layers for model skull construction.
Fig. 4/39. Model skull tightly glued with Araldite.

Model Skulls

The human skull is made up of a combination of materials (C), i.e. the hard (H) material of the outer table, the soft (S) thick cancellous middle portion and the hard (H) inner table resembling the outer table (fig. 4/37, 3).

The bones of the human skull are difficult to simulate due to their biochemical and histological composition. However, it is possible to construct something resembling the bone of the human skull in respect of function and morphology by making the thin outer and inner layers out of Palacos and the soft thick middle layer out of plasticine (fig. 4/38).

The experimental model skulls were made of the same materials as used in my previous experimental model, i.e. with plasticine as soft material and with Palacos as hard material. Palacos plates, 1–2 mm thick, were made for the outer and inner tables, and 3–5 mm of plasticine was used for the middle portion, the layers being glued tightly together with Araldite (fig. 4/39).

The depressed fractures (fig. 4/40) were produced with a pointed impactor (fig. 4/41) used in a previous experimental study, and the experi-

---

Fig. 4/36. A shattering fracture (**B**) and (**C**) was the only result, even when a pointed impactor (**A**) was used. P = Pointed impactor; B = direction of impact.

Fig. 4/37. Fracturing of different materials.

4/40

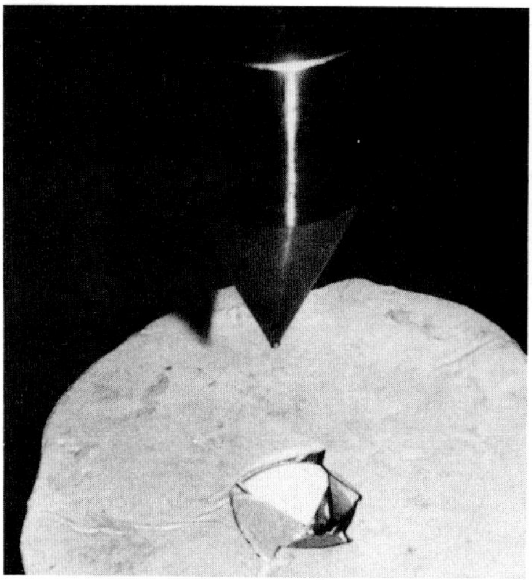

4/4

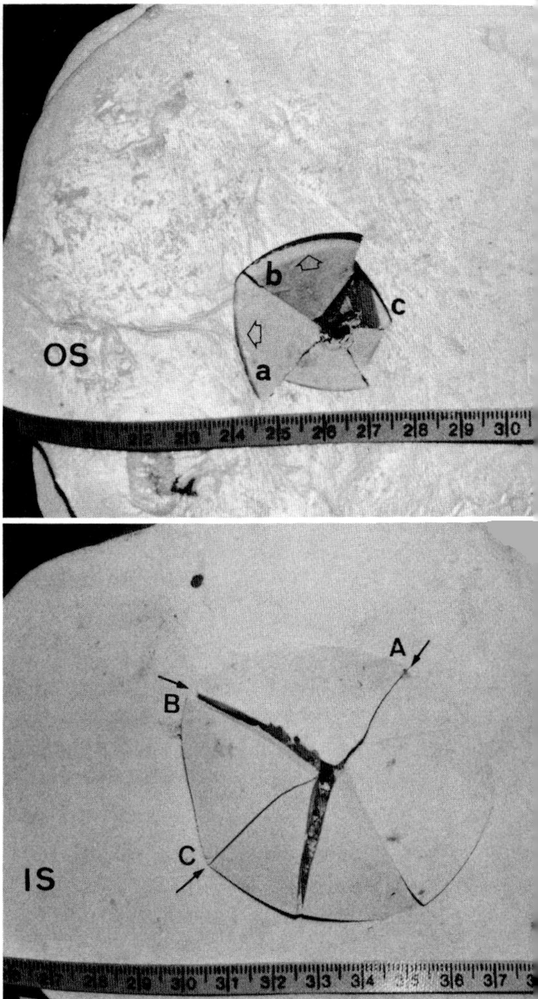

4/

Fig. 4/40. Pointed impactor and resulting depressed fracture of the model skull.

Fig. 4/41. A Smaller depressed fracture of the outer side (OS). **B** Larger depressed fracture of the inner side (IS).

mental procedures in this study were the same. Depressed fractures were produced in all these model plates.

It was noteworthy that they all showed a larger fracture of the inner side than of the outer side (fig. 4/40) resembling the reaction of the human skull.

The X-ray picture of the depressed fracture shows a larger fracture shadow (ABC) on the inner side and smaller fracture (abc) on the outer

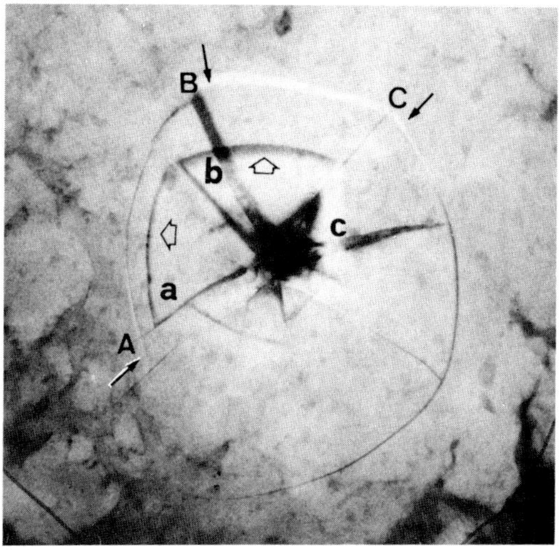

4/42

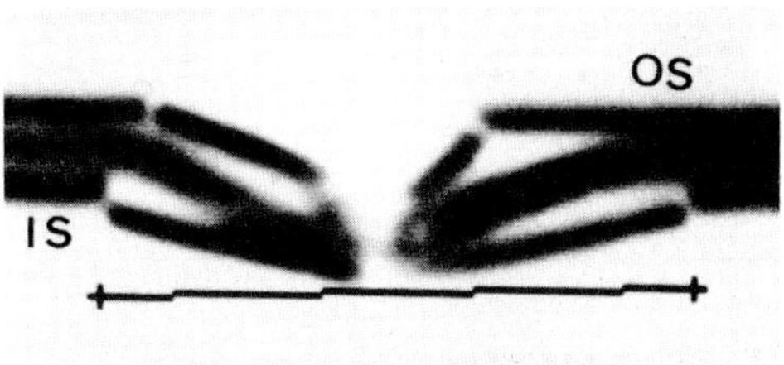

4/43A

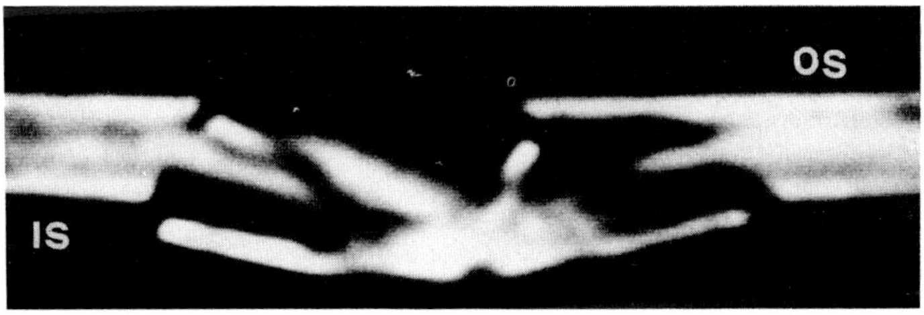

4/43B

Fig. 4/42. X-ray image. Clear visualisation of the larger fracture of the inner layer than of the outer layer.

Fig. 4/43A, B. CT findings. OS < IS.

layer, and many fracture fragments (fig. 4/42). A CT scan (lateral view) clearly visualised each layer (especially the soft middle layer), and the typical inverted V form of the depressed fracture of the model skull (fig. 4/43A, B).

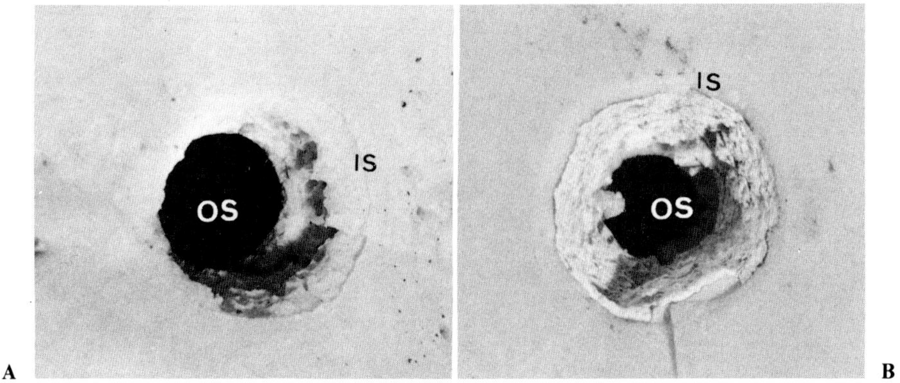

Fig. 4/44. A Human skull. **B** Experimental model.

These experimental model skull bones always showed a larger fracture of the inner than of the outer side, the same morphological features as in human skulls at low velocities of 2–5 kN (fig. 4/15).

I have carried out a comparative study with high velocities. For these comparative studies, I used a 22-calibre pistol at a distance of 3 m, equivalent to about 130 J with 22 long rifle ammunition. 5 human skulls and 5 experimental model skulls were tested. The behavior of the fracture fragments at high velocity is quite different from that at low velocity; they shattered into powder and disappeared (so-called perforating fracture). However, the small-area high velocity impacts also showed the typical inverted V form of the depressed fracture (fig. 4/44) in these bone models and in the human skulls.

Discussion

Travelling at high speed in a crouched position, skiers often suffer direct head injuries from contact with a variety of obstacles, especially depressed fractures with or without brain lesions/hemorrhages, and these require immediate surgical treatment [39].

A typical type of head injury, namely depressed fracture, was found in 84% of all skiing accidents requiring surgical intervention. During operation, it was always found that the fracture of the inner table was larger

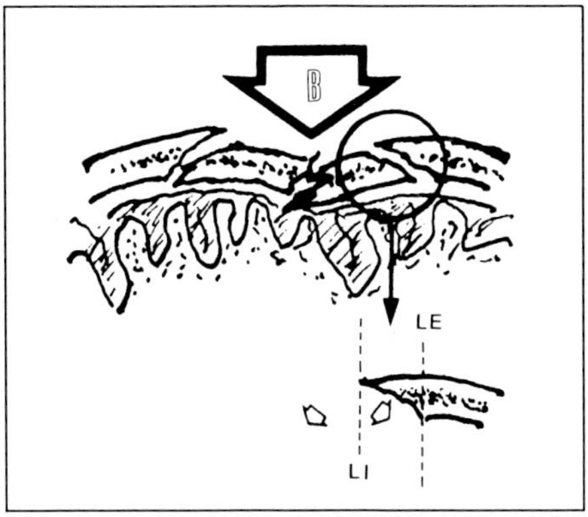

Fig. 4/45. Illustration of a typical depressed skull fructure. B = Direction of impact.

than that of the outer table, and this made reduction difficult (fig. 4/45) [45, 49].

First, I carried out an experimental study of the relation between impact forces and depressed fractures. This confirmed that a low force applied to a small area results in depressed fractures, and a high velocity results in perforating fractures. Secondly, I found the same characteristic morphology, that is, a larger fracture of the inner table than of the outer table, as is found clinically. Nobody has yet explained the mechanism of production of these characteristic morphological effects and structures. The human skull is made up of 3 functionally distinct morphological layers, the hard outer and inner tables and the soft, thick cancellous middle portion.

I suspected that the mechanism of production of this type of depressed fracture must be due to the combination of functional morphological structures.

After experimental studies on soft and hard materials, I constructed the models of skull bone and produced depressed fractures using the previous experimental methods. The application of small-area impacts resulted in depressed fractures with the same morphological characteristics as in real human skulls [49].

Based on the results of these experiments, I can explain the mechanism of production of depressed fractures as follows [43, 45, 49]. *First stage:* the skull sustains the force of the impact first on the hard outer table, and this causes a linear fracture. *Second stage:* the energy spreads out into the soft,

4/46 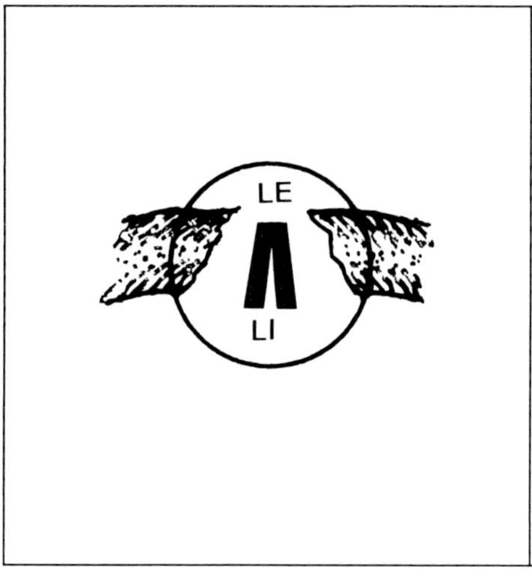

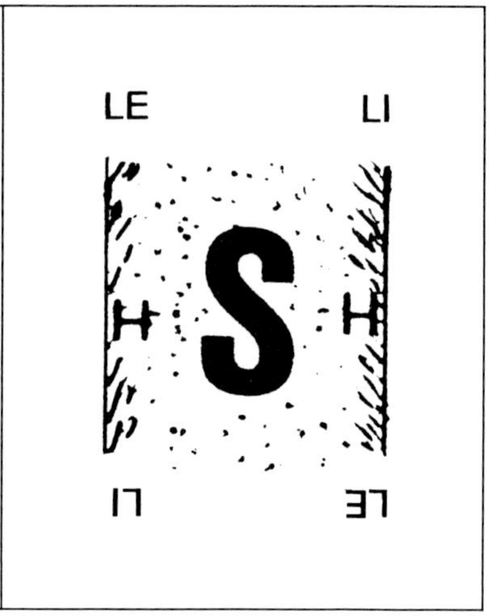 4/47

Fig. 4/46. Typical form of the depressed fracture.

Fig. 4/47. Morphology of the functional structure of the human skull. LE = Lamina externa; LI = lamina interna; H = hard layer; S = soft thick portion.

thick middle layer. *Third stage:* the remaining energy reaches the hard inner table and causes a larger fracture than in the outer table.

I call the clinically typical form, of the depressed fracture the inverted V fracture (fig. 4/46), and the functional structure of the human skull the HSH layer (fig. 4/47).

Four main points were observed in these experiments on human skulls and on model skulls: (1) When the direct force applied was small, depressed fractures occurred at low velocity and perforating fractures at high speed. (2) The fracture of the inner table was always larger than that of the outer table, resulting from the directions of the kinetic energies, and this is called the typical inverted V form. (3) The type of inverted V form of the depressed fracture does not depend upon the velocity. (4) These depressed fractures only happen in HSH structures which resemble human skulls.

These depressed skull fractures may require surgery [3, 26, 29, 32, 39, 49].

5 First Aid and Immediate Treatment

As already mentioned in the chapter on the causes of accidents, head injuries during skiing are often serious and sometimes fatal.

A well-organised three-way system of cooperation (fig. 5/1) results in optimal care of the patients, preventing brain stem compression before irreversible damage has occurred (case 33, fig. 3/56).

Ski-lift personnel, first aid services and transportation employees in skiing regions must be trained to help in cases of acute head injuries, so that optimal team work is assured. Every year the slope layouts are improved and faster pistes are provided for the skiers, resulting in increased accident risks.

First Aid at Accident Site

As indicated elsewhere, it would be best if more than 3 persons were to ski together in case an accident should occur. This should ensure optimal functioning of first aid, as illustrated by figure 5/2:

(1) Skier No. 2 (fig. 6/1) should immediately stick his skis and those of the injured person crosswise into the snow above the patient, so that the skiers following behind can navigate around the accident site (fig. 5/3). Until help arrives, the patient (if unconscious) is to be placed in a sideways position and checked for free breathing. Where there is an open wound with heavy bleeding, any kind of compression material available (e.g. cap, gloves) should be applied to prevent hypovolemic shock from excessive loss of blood.

(2) The third skier (fig. 6/1) must proceed immediately to the nearest service station (for instance a ski-lift station where a phone or radio is located) and inform them so that the rescue service can be notified to provide assistance (fig. 5/2).

(3) The rescue service must bc informed about the accident by phone or shortwave radio at once.

5/1

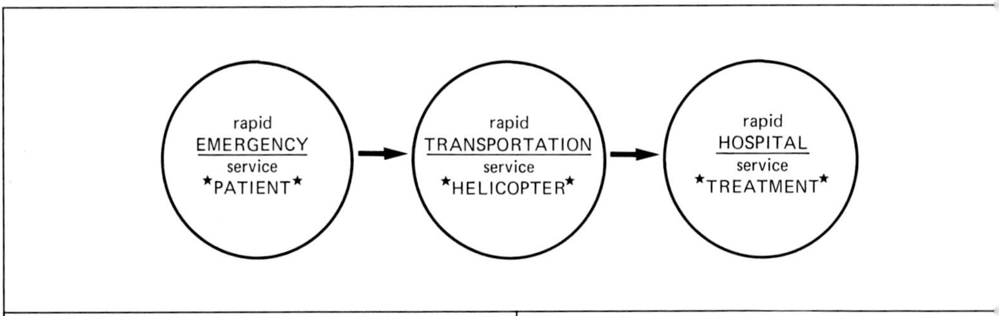

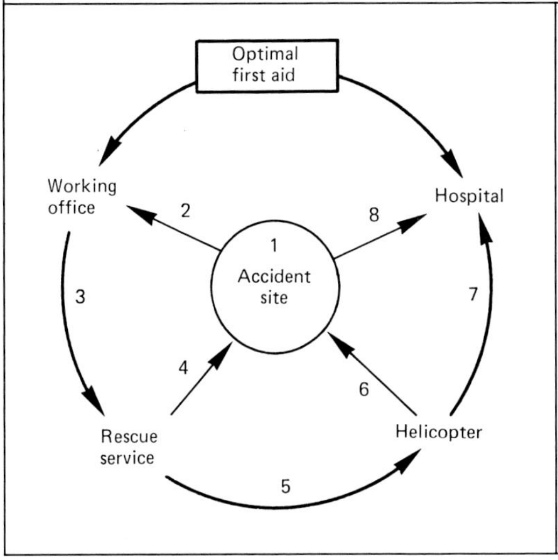

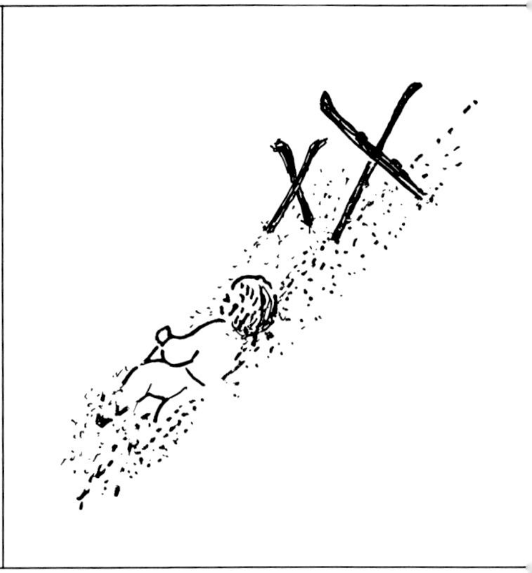

5/2 5/3

Fig. 5/1. Optimal first aid service system.
Fig. 5/2. Illustration of optimal first aid.
Fig. 5/3. Two pairs of crossed skis stuck in the snow.

(4) A rescue squad, equipped to assist (with, e.g., compression bandages), must proceed to the accident site immediately and determine as far as possible how severely the patient is injured. Additional rescue service personnel should then be notified by shortwave radio to arrange for prompt transport, preferably by helicopter. The helicopter service is well organised in this canton (Graubünden) and is prepared for the immediate transport of severely injured skiers. There is geographical co-ordination of their activities, with command stations located in Samedan and in Untervaz.

(5) The rescue personnel are responsible for immediate despatch of the helicopter and notification of the arrival time at the scene of the accident,

A 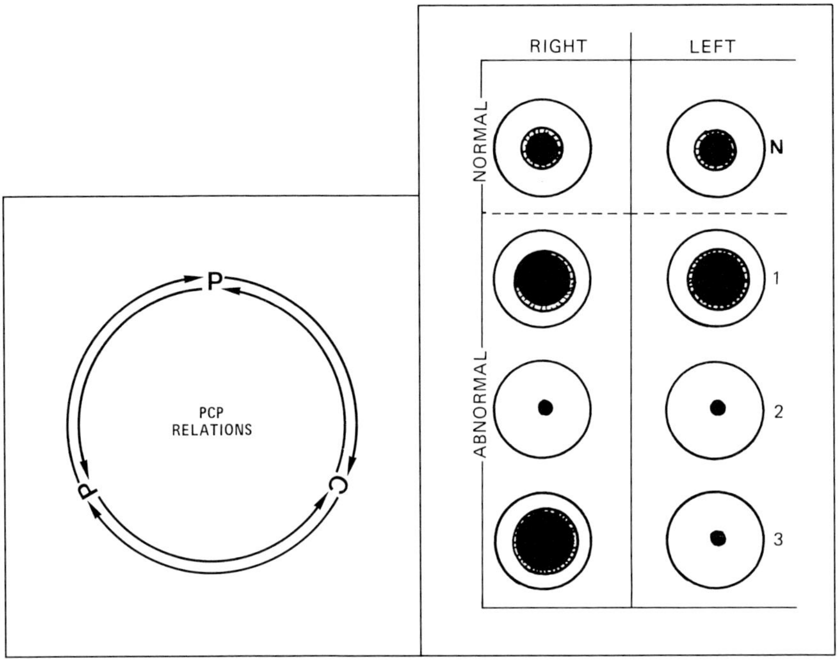 B

Fig. 5/4. 'PCP' test. **A** PCP circle of relations. P = Pupil and pain ; C = consciousness. **B** Conditions of the pupils. N = Normal pupils; 1 = 'hopeless' pupils; 2 = 'hopeful' pupils; 3 = 'surgical' pupils.

and they should stay in contact with the rescue squad to ensure that appropriate assistance is rendered until it arrives. In order to help patients with head injuries, the rescue squad personnel should have some basic medical training, to be able to perform the 'PCP' (fig. 5/4) and 'ENT' tests (fig. 5/5).

The PCP test method is simple and straightforward, and the findings are very important for the prognosis of the patient's recovery. No medical instruments are required for the PCP test. The results of the PCP test are interrelated (fig. 5/4A).

First, the patient's pupils must be checked and then it is possible to determine the prognosis, whether 'hopeless' or 'hopeful' or 'doubtful' (fig. 5/4B):

N, normal pupils: Prompt symmetrical reaction to sunlight with moderate-sized pupils. Disturbance of consciousness: none or slight, with brisk response to pain (fig. 5/4B, N).

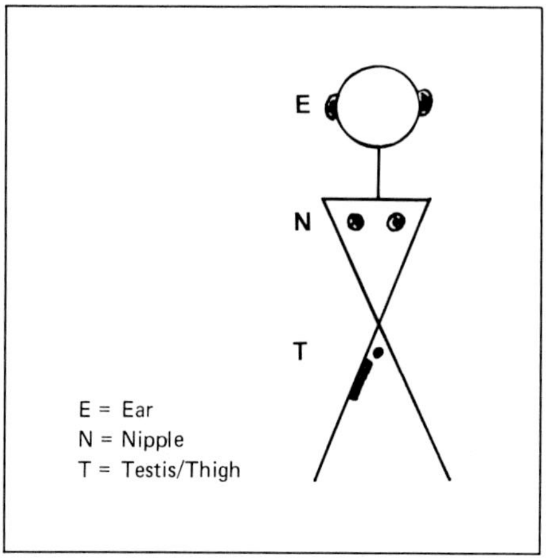

Fig. 5/5. Simple 'ENT' method for response to pain.

1, hopeless pupils: Fixed dilated pupils mean a 'hopeless' condition due to direct or indirect brainstem damage. No response to pain or decerebrate rigidity response with comatose state (fig. 5/4B, 1).

2, hopeful pupils: Irritable pupils mean a 'hopeful' condition of the patient. They derive from intracranial parasympathetic stimulation due to brain edema. The prognosis is good. Slight to moderate disturbance of consciousness with prompt response to pain (purposive movement of all 4 limbs). Anisocoria may develop occasionally (fig. 5/4B, 2).

3, surgical pupils (anisocoria) (fig. 5/4B, 3): They indicate incipient brain stem compression on one side, usually due to acute hemorrhage. Deep unconsciousness usually accompanied by contralateral motor weakness. Fixed dilated pupils (hopeless pupils) rapidly develop. Before this occurs, optimal first aid, rapid transfer to neurosurgical department, and immediate surgical decompressive treatment are absolutely essential. In such a case, the rescue squad must insist on immediate transport. During the interim an occasional check of the pupils is recommended. If fixed dilated pupils develop, surgical decompression is necessary within 1 h, otherwise the chance of survival for adults is very poor.

Normal or hopeful pupils with weak or no response to pain in the limbs indicate possible spine damage.

In order to limit the danger of secondary damage, particularly in cases of unstable spinal fracture with or without paralysis, it should be checked

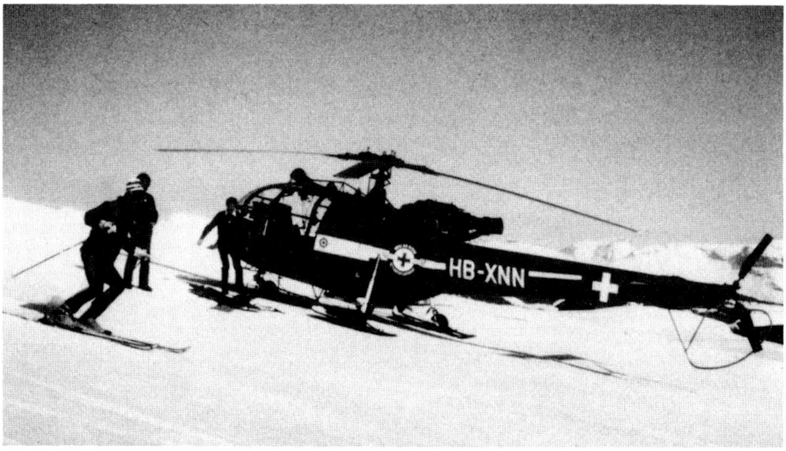

Fig. 5/6. Air-rescue service should always be at the alert (REGA/Switzerland).

prior to transportation, by the movement responses to painful stimuli, whether cervical, thoracic or lumbar lesions are involved. There is a simple method for this, the 'ENT' tests (fig. 5/5). The 'ENT' tests are, of course, only indicated for unconscious patients and should be performed as follows:

E (ear): First, pinch the ear. If movement of all 4 limbs results, no paralysis is present. If the movement of the upper limbs is nil or only slight, there is possibly a cervical lesion.

N (nipple): An area very sensitive to pain. If there is no movement response of one side of the body (arm and leg), then a brain lesion is possible. If there is no movement of the lower limbs (both legs), there is suspicion of a lumbar or lower thoracic spine lesion.

T (testis/thigh): The test is carried out by pinching not the testicles themselves (women – inside of thigh) but the skin covering them. If both legs do not move, a thoracolumbar lesion could be possible.

If the movement response of the 4 limbs is weak (tetraparesis), to avoid secondary damage, very careful transportation is necessary, with prompt admission to hospital, because urgent treatment of the suspected cervical spine lesions is essential.

Until transport arrives, the patient should be cautiously moved from the slope, so that it is free for skiing again. If possible, the patient should be moved to a spot near which a helicopter is able to land.

If the patient vomits, or bleeding from the nose or mouth is found, the patient must be placed in a sideways position and checked for free breathing.

(6) The helicopter service (REGA/Switzerland, fig. 5/6) should always be in a state of readiness. The air rescue service is well equipped to provide emergency aid, primarily for disorders of respiration and circulation. First aid is often provided by medical assistants. Severely injured patients with respiratory distress should be intubated at the scene of the accident and receive an infusion during transportation.

(7) Before or at the time of departure, the hospital should be notified of the expected arrival time, so that the necessary preparations can be made before the patient is admitted.

(8) It is desirable for the hospital to receive the following additional information before the departure: extent of injuries, age of the patient, whether intubated or not, whether there are any other injuries.

In cases of open head injuries, with or without accompanying disturbance of consciousness or neurological deficits, the patient should be transferred directly to a neurosurgical hospital, where any depressed fracture can be verified radiologically. This would require immediate surgery, and is often the case in skiing accidents.

At the scene of the accident the patient may complain of increasingly severe migrainous headache (at the site of impact) but have no impairment of consciousness, due to the fact that accidents on hard or icy slopes may often cause a linear parietotemporal fracture of the skull, which may result in incipient epidural hematoma (with a so-called lucid interval). If the patient complains of nausea (with vomiting), he should be urgently transferred to a neurosurgical department before he develops signs of brain stem compression.

Immediate Treatment

This means the treatment undertaken within 24 h. After a thorough examination in the emergency room, it is important to decide whether treatment should be conservative or surgical (fig. 5/7).

The indications mainly relate to the type of injury (open/closed) and to the findings of neuroradiology and computed tomography (depressed fracture, hematoma, malignant edema, etc.) [27].

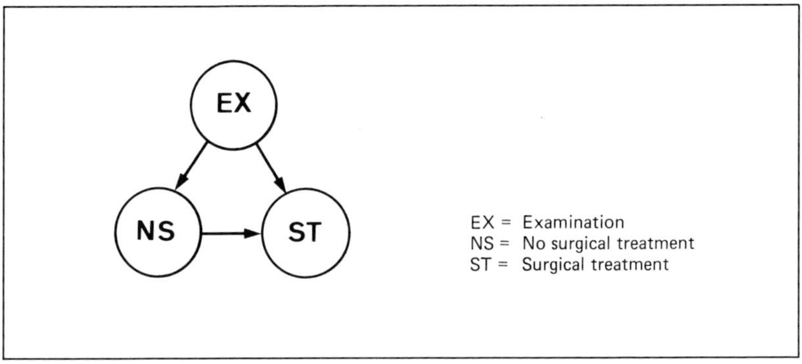

Fig. 5/7. Immediate treatment at the hospital.

Conservative Therapy

In cases where the score on the Glasgow scale is above 8 (brain contusion), careful circulatory and neurological monitoring is necessary for 24 h. Nonsurgical treatment is considered for patients with severe contusion of the brain and having a Glasgow score below 7. These patients should be intubated and an epidural intracranial pressure gauge inserted for continuous monitoring of brain pressure.

Between January 1980 and July 1981, the brain pressures of 27 patients were measured, 23 of whom had head injuries. The necessity of measuring the intracranial pressure was indicated whenever the Glasgow score was below 7 points without craniotomy/craniectomy being required [14].

20 cases underwent epidural procedures, and in 7 cases a ventricular drain was inserted. Measurements were carried out on-line with epidural screws and a mini-transducer. In cases with ventricular drainage, the measuring was done at intervals using a double three-way valve. During that time, the therapy consisted of intubation with hyperventilation at a PA_{CO_2} of 25–30 mm Hg (27 cases), forced diuresis with furosemide (27 cases), dexamethasone (26 cases), and relaxation with curare preparations. The patients were relaxed only to 'tractability' (25 cases), and received mannitol 0.5–2 g/kg (14 cases), barbiturates (thiopental 15–30 mg/kg, 9 cases) and therapeutic CSF drainage (8 cases). Despite all these conservative measures, the intracranial pressure rose more than *30 mm Hg* (i.e. deterioration of condition), making immediate radical surgical treatment necessary, namely a large craniectomy, opening of the dura, removal of necrotic/hemorrhagic

5/8

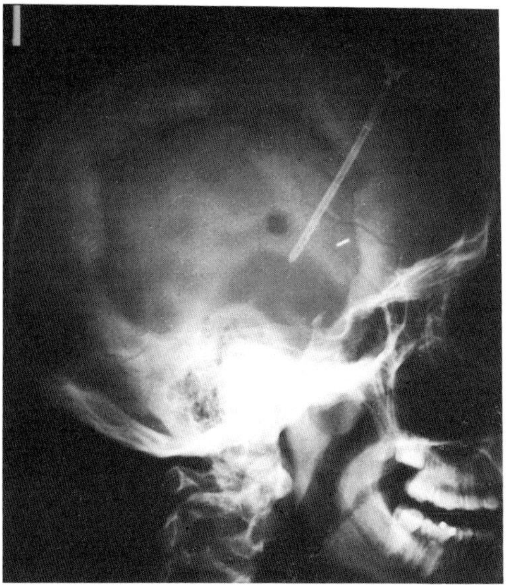

5/9

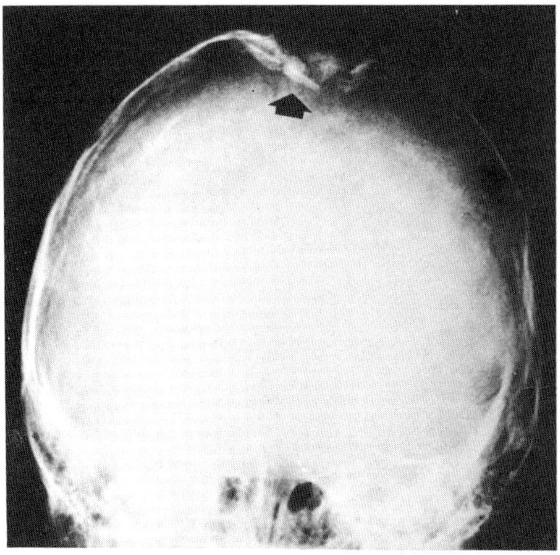

Fig. 5/8. Large decompressive craniectomy with ventricular drainage.
Fig. 5/9. Open depressed fracture which required immediate surgical treatment.

brain tissue and open ventricular drainage. If closing the scalp is impossible because of brain swelling, then a frontal lobectomy or temporal lobe resection is indicated. This radical surgical treatment is usually successful in children and young patients.

Immediate Surgical Treatment

This must be performed within 24 h.

(a) Radical decompressive surgery: Where preceding intensive conservative therapy is unsuccessful and there is incipient brain stem compression, radical surgery is performed, namely craniectomy, removal of hemorrhagic/necrotic brain tissue (even frontal resection), loosening of the dura and open ventricular drainage (fig. 5/8).

(b) Open head injuries: Depressed fractures with or without brain damage are typical injuries in skiing accidents. If during examination (palpation) an open depressed fracture is detected, immediate surgical treatment is required (fig. 5/9).

5/11

5/10

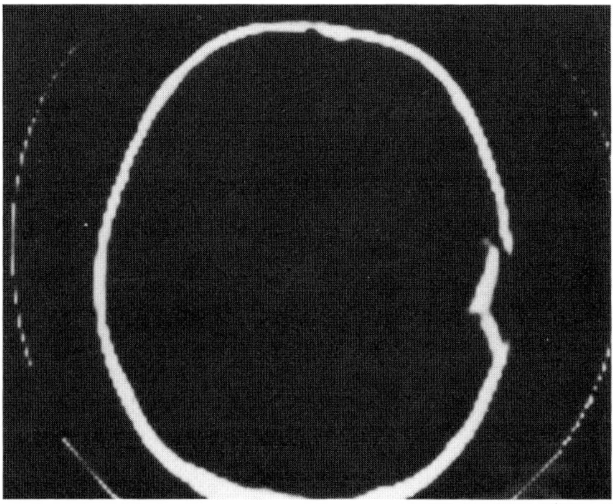

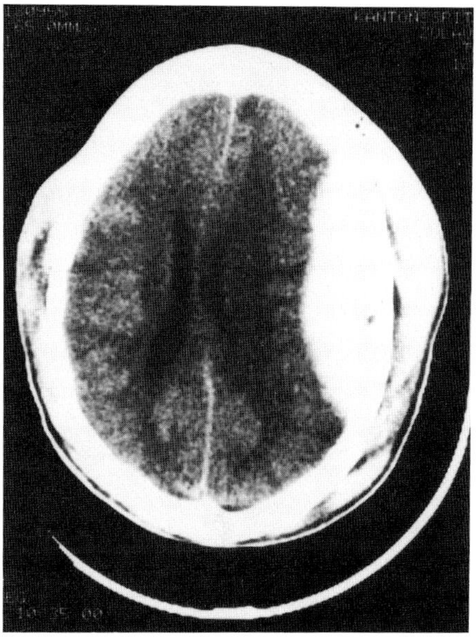

Fig. 5/10. CT scan. Closed depressed (motor area) fracture with neurological signs (paresis) requiring immediate operation.

Fig. 5/11. Acute epidural hematoma which resulted in brain stem compression a few hours after accident occurred.

(c) Closed depressed fracture with neurological signs: Revelation by radiology or CT scan of a depressed fracture in the parietotemporal region in association with neurological deficits (fig. 5/10), especially motor or speech disorders, indicates immediate decompressive surgery [63].

(d) Epidural hematoma: Linear fracture in the parietotemporal area with rapid deterioration of consciousness, caused by an acute epidural hematoma as confirmed by CT scan, necessitates an immediate surgical decompressive procedure before a brain stem syndrome develops. All skull fractures, particularly where a linear parietotemporal fracture has been confirmed radiologically, require strict 24-hour surveillance, as there is a danger of symptoms of acute brain stem compression caused by an acute epidural hematoma (fig. 5/11).

(e) Acute contusion hematoma (fig. 5/12): This first causes no significant signs of pressure on the brain, and can be more or less controlled by conservative treatment. Later, there is rapid deterioration in the patient's

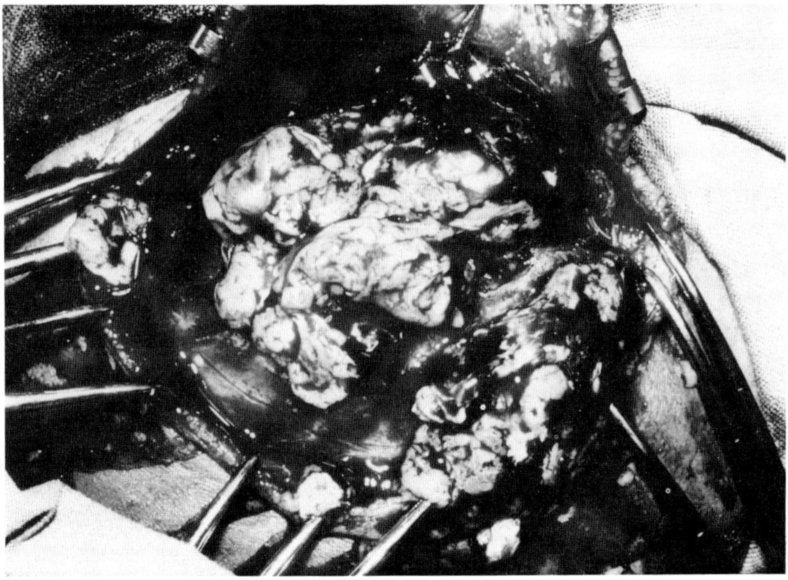

Fig. 5/12. Acute contusion hematoma (finding at operation).

condition, usually due to malignant edema from the contusion. Radical decompressive surgery is indicated, but the prognosis is usually poor, particularly for adults and elderly patients.

Surgical measures required after more than 24 h have elapsed (subacute phase) are not under consideration here.

6 Prevention

Generally speaking, all activities involving speed (like flying, driving a car, or skiing) are connected with a risk of accident, because effects of speed may cause injuries. The ski slopes, just like the roads, are public highways and can be used by everyone without restriction, and thus many accidents occur. At peak hours or weekends there is much more traffic on the ski slopes than on the roads. When driving a car, speed restrictions apply and traffic lanes with prohibition of passing exist, and there are other strictly enforced regulations. In contrast, there are no actual regulations applying on the ski slopes. Children and adults, women and men may ski without needing a permit. As a result, although skiing is enjoyable and healthy, many serious accidents occur each year, unfortunately.

With the ever-increasing numbers participating in this most popular sport, there is a pressing need for a thorough accident prevention programme.

As in traffic accidents, in skiing we can differentiate between accidents caused by the injured person and those caused by someone else. For the prevention of these accidents, *indirect* or *direct* measures must be taken.

Indirect Preventive Measures

Personal Aspects

Lack of physical fitness [20], poor skiing technique, overtiredness, alcohol consumption and so on can play an important part in causing accidents. Untrained skiers certainly suffer more accidents than trained ones.

Well-trained skiers in good physical condition have fewer accidents than less well-trained skiers. In particular, excessive alcohol consumption will increase the risk of accidents, just like when driving a car.

For example, a 23-year-old male (case 36) was skiing under the influence of alcohol when he tumbled over a wall about 3 m high and

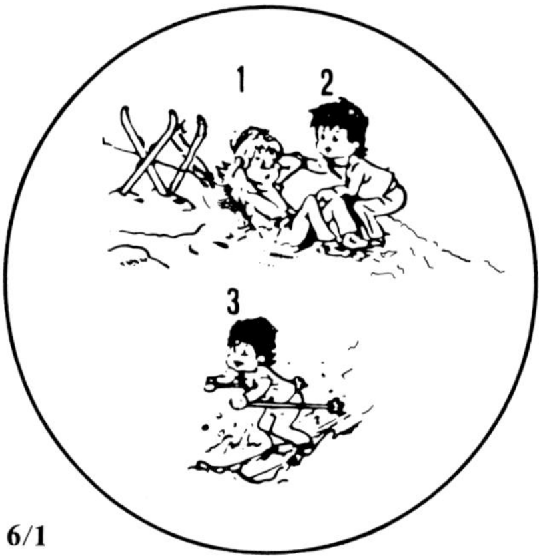

6/1

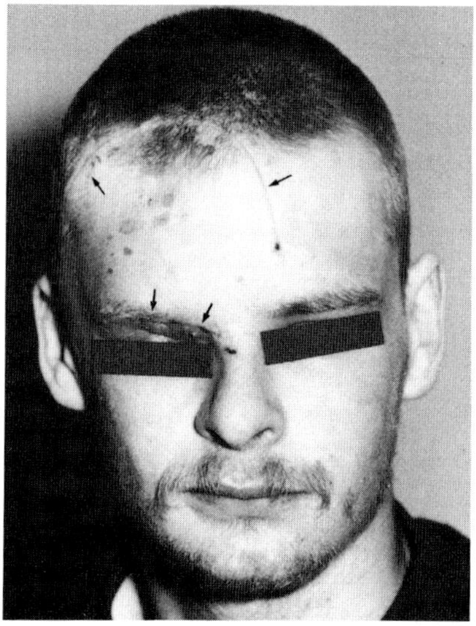

6/2

Fig. 6/1. Schematic illustration of accident and immediate measures to be taken. 1 = Patient; 2 = lookout; 3 = messenger.

Fig. 6/2. The patient shown after operation.

finished up in a garden fence. He immediately lost consciousness. On admission to hospital he was somnolent with alcohol on his breath. He suffered a frontobasal fracture and a fracture of the nasal bone.

Accidental Aspects

Skiing as a recreation should be enjoyed at leisure and with friends or family.

It is best if more than three skiers go out together (fig. 6/1). Then, if an accident occurs, one can remain with the patient and prevent other fast or careless skiers from crashing into him, while the third can erect a warning sign of skis (fig. 6/1) and either go himself for help or send another skier.

If the injured person in figure 2/3 had not been alone, this tragic outcome would most likely have been avoided by the availability of help and by giving other skiers the alarm. This case illustrates clearly that children in particular should not be allowed to ski alone.

It is not rare for an injured skier (particularly one who is unconscious) to be discovered by someone passing by, and then what happened to cause the accident remains unknown.

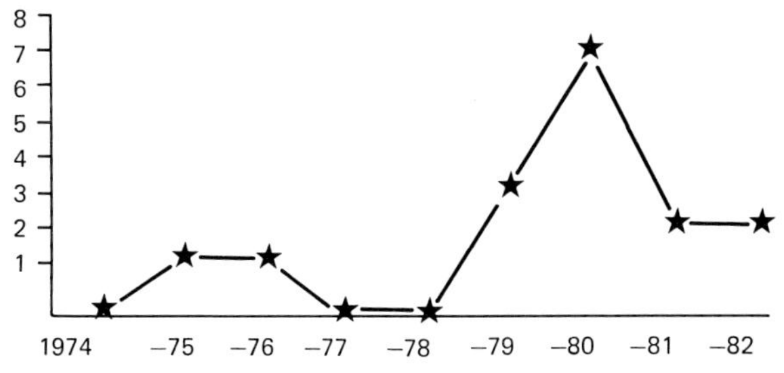

Fig. 6/3. Distribution of the fatal cases.

For example, the unconscious patient (case 32), was found on the open ski slope by passing skiers. He had been skiing alone. The cause of the accident is unknown. He suffered an extended open laceration of the right eyelid (fig. 6/2) with a comminuted depressed frontobasal fracture on the right, and underwent immediate operation. He still complained of double vision at discharge.

Natural Aspects

Weather (sunshine, cloudy, snowing, etc.) and ski slope conditions (powder snow or hard and icy, etc.) have a great effect on the risk of accidents [20, 28]. A hard or icy slope is very dangerous and can give rise to severe head injuries even from minor falls. Ski slope conditions vary with the time of day and the time of year, and with changes in temperature, especially in February and March, when the snow is usually hard in the morning but heavier in the afternoon sunshine. Conditions on southern slopes and northern slopes vary accordingly. Long skis are more suitable for hard or icy slopes, while short skis are easier on wet slopes. An insufficient amount of snow on the ski slope is also dangerous and may occasionally lead to accidents [57].

In the 1979/1980 ski season, many severe head injuries occurred due to insufficient snow on the slopes (fig. 6/3) and 7 of these were fatal.

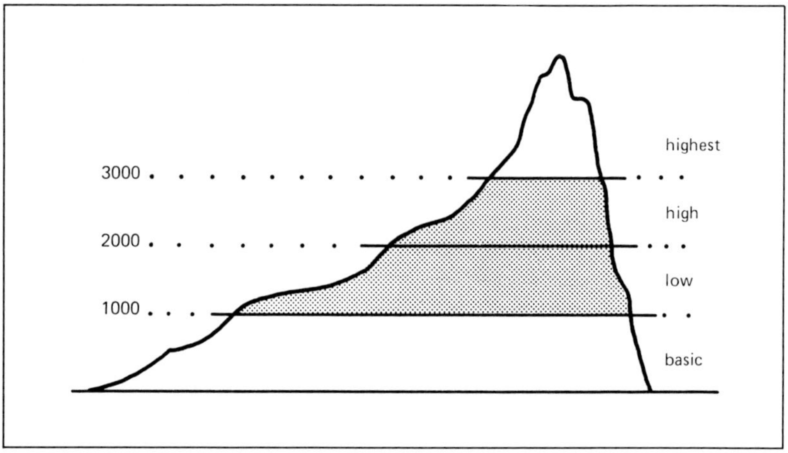

Fig. 6/4. Altitude of ski slopes.

During snowfall and fog, there will be poor visibility and disorientation on the slopes, which again may cause accidents, mainly due to slipping or sliding.

In the Alps (from Austria to France) most ski slopes are located at altitudes between 1,000 and 3,000 m. There are 4 categories (fig. 6/4) as follows:

The *basic* altitude ski slope is short and not steep and is used mostly by local skiers. It often runs through forests with many natural and artificial obstacles, which demand care to be exercised to avoid accidents.

The *low* altitude slope is better for skiing than the basic slope. Although it also has many obstacles, the snow conditions are better; it is usually steeper and located amongst alpine huts.

The *high* altitude slope is usually ideal due to the natural conditions of the Alps; there are no trees and no artificial obstacles on it.

The *highest* altitude slope is rarely used during the winter. It is called the 'summer ski slope'. Often cold, cloudy weather with strong winds prevails and the low oxygen at such altitudes leads to dizziness and unreliable physical responses, which cause dangerous accidents.

The choice of the altitude of the slope to use depends on the time of day (morning or afternoon), day of the week (weekday or weekend), month of the year, and the prevailing weather conditions. The choice is important for the indirect prevention of accidents.

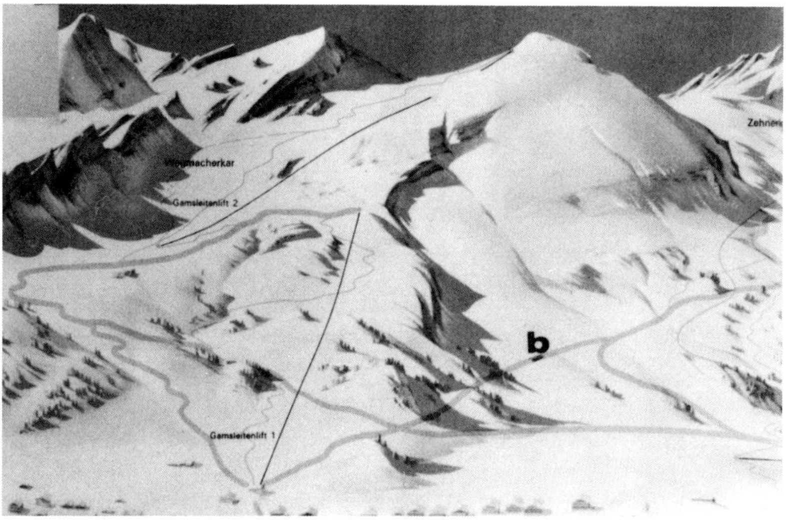

Fig. 6/5. Blue (b), easy slope.

Technical Aspects

Whether a skier is good or not, and whether he is experienced or a beginner, makes little difference when it comes to head injuries. The adjustment of the bindings cannot be done alone but should be performed by an expert, because skier, boots, skis and bindings form a functional unit, in which each part has to fit. Periodic checks of the equipment and, in particular, proper adjustment of the safety bindings are of the utmost importance [34, 53]. It is well to remember that a slack adjustment, with quick release of the bindings, also represents a considerable risk factor [9, 21]. From time to time boots and skis must be modified to conform with the most recent technical advances. Notice boards and information signs near ski-lifts and cable cars provide clear information on the various descents, their degree of difficulty and the snow conditions. Beginners should always choose an easy slope, i.e. a blue slope (fig. 6/5).

Traffic Aspects

The ski-lift service should be discontinued when there is heavy snowfall or foggy conditions or strong winds.

Despite the improved T-bars now in use on ski-lifts, more attention should be paid to their design, because they still cause many head injuries,

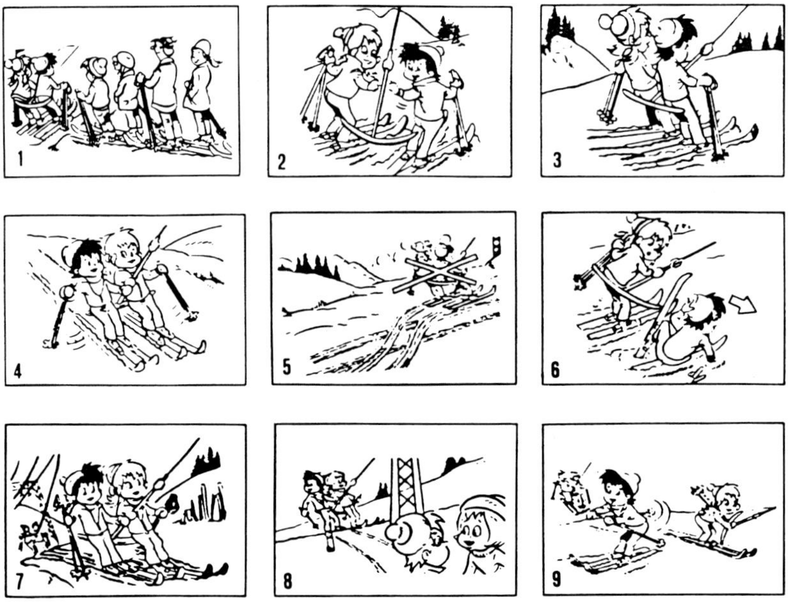

Fig. 6/6. Using ski-lift und T-bar.

particularly to children. I have seen many patients with head injuries caused by collisions with ski-lift bars [46].

The following 9 points (illustrated in figure 6/6) relate to the prevention of accidents when using ski-lift T-bars. These are the recommendations of the German Ski Federation (DSV) [61]. Especially at the weekend and during school vacations, there are long queues of skiers waiting to use the T-bars of ski-lifts (fig. 6/7).

(1) Queuing – Stand in an orderly line, for disc lifts in single file, and for T-bar lifts in pairs, in order to avoid backups and unnecessary waiting time. Note whether it is a self-service lift or one with an attendant. Only if it is a self-service lift may you catch hold of the disc or bar.

(2) Getting on – Move quickly toward the entrance gate and, holding both ski sticks with the outside hand, face toward the inside, so that you can grab the tow bar with your free hand.

(3) Starting – Do not sit on the T-bar. Remain standing, lean lightly against the bar and let yourself be pushed. Sliding steps in the direction of movement will facilitate starting.

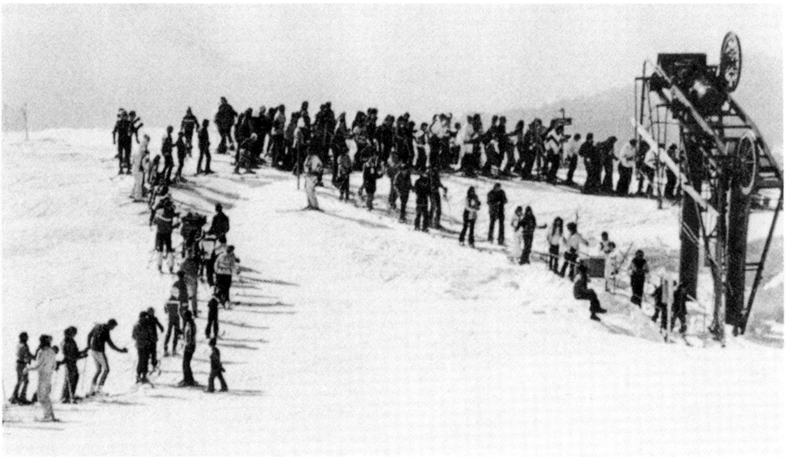

Fig. 6/7. Long queue for ski-lift.

(4) Conduct during trip – Keep your skis slightly open and with an even weight distribution on both skis. So as to keep a good balance, do not lean toward the outside or toward your partner.
(5) Stay in your track – Your skis should remain in the tracks. Do not 'slalom' or get off prematurely, otherwise you will endanger yourself and others.
(6) Behavior after a fall – An attempt must be made to get off the tracks immediately; those behind have little chance to take evasive action.
(7) Preparation for getting off – Get ready in good time. Take care that the towbar is not caught in your clothing.
(8) Getting off – Get off quickly, allow the T-bar to continue moving in the same direction and do not push it aside carelessly.
(9) Leaving the exit gate – Leave the exit at once to make room for the skiers behind, so that no collisions occur and you avoid being hit by one of the moving T-bars.

Carelessness or slow reactions when getting on the ski-lift T-bar often results in skull fractures (from impact of the T-bar), as shown in cases 16 and 17 [18, 46].

The rules of behavior (German version) [62] are contained in the 'Ski Atlas 1983', and the Swiss version is in the 'Drive for safety in sport' [53]

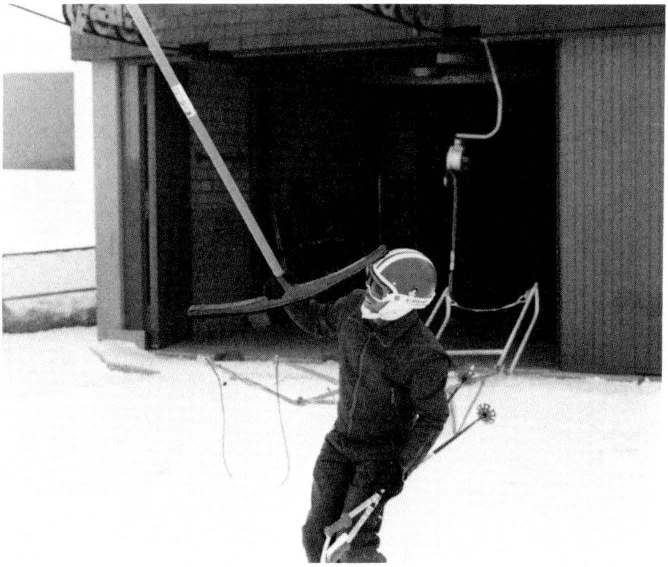

Fig. 6/8. Helmet prevents head injuries.

and is already displayed at some ski-lift stations. At the start of every winter season, they should be brought to the attention of those for whom they are intended (particularly children and young people), since it has been proven statistically that there is a definite relation between rule violation and the incidence of accidents. In addition, maintenance and servicing of ski-lift systems should be improved and the technology brought up to date by, for instance, introducing TV monitoring. Then, if an incident takes place, the supervisory personnel can take immediate action. On the other hand, appropriate personal equipment (wearing a safety helmet for instance), (fig. 6/8) can improve individual protection. This is the way to prevent direct head injuries from ski-lift accidents.

The safety use of a ski-lift demands some knowledge of the behavior required and the dangers involved (indirect prevention) [46, 61].

The rules of behavior (fig. 6/6) should be read by all skiers at the beginning of every winter season, and they should be followed. I recommend the wearing of a safety helmet (fig. 6/8) instead of a cap (direct prevention), particularly by children and young skiers. This represents an effective and sensible method of prevention of head injuries.

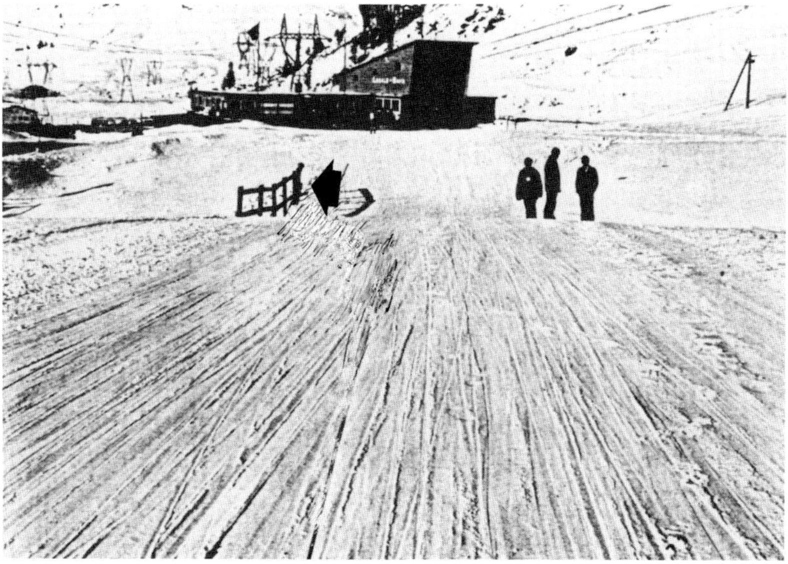

Fig. 6/9. Collision with this wooden fence resulted in fatal head injury.

As all skiers move from the top to the bottom of the slope (as in a one-way street), direct forehead to forehead collisions are normally impossible. Such collisions take place only on crossing ski slopes, for which reason all crossing of slopes should be made safe by means of overpasses.

Furthermore, better signs giving information about danger spots and poor visibility and advising the skier to reduce speed should be placed on all slopes.

Particularly dangerous areas on the slopes should be marked and cushioned fencing installed. Wooden or metal fences are very dangerous, as illustrated by the case which resulted in death (fig. 6/9).

The installation of a sign has little meaning for children and young skiers, as have street signs, unless they have been taught to obey them at home or in school.

Social Aspects

The general public should be made aware of the medical fact that the nerve tissue of the central nervous system are unable to regenerate, and thus differ from bones for instance. Organic damage to the central nervous sys-

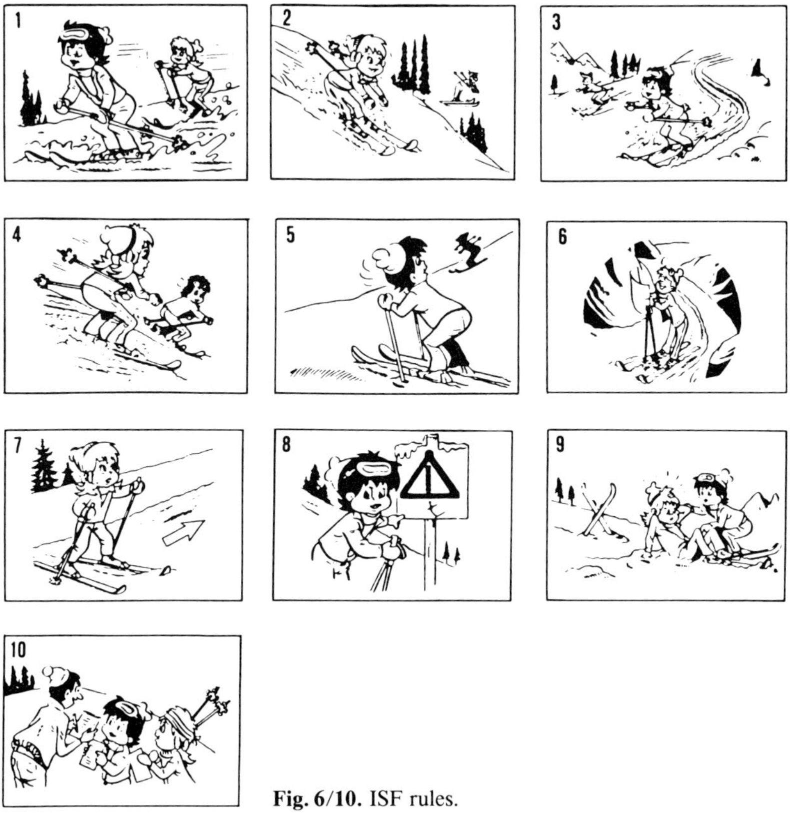

Fig. 6/10. ISF rules.

tem therefore leads to irreversible functional disorders. In contrast to road accidents, it is often impossible to establish exactly who is guilty in ski slope accidents, because official ski slope regulations have never been drawn up or widely accepted. The introduction of such slope regulations and the publication of clear rules regarding behavior on the slopes is just as necessary as informing the skiers about accident prevention. The international organisation of cable cars and ski-lifts, with the intention of preventing accidents on ski slopes as far as possible, has adopted a code of safety rules and is asking that they be obeyed [11]. These rules of behavior were drawn up by the legal committee of the International Ski Federation (ISF) and accepted by the ISF Congress on May 20, 1967 in Beirut (fig. 6/10) [61]. Like every other sport, skiing has some risks for those who do it, but there are also responsibilities in civil and criminal law.

The following 10 points of the slope rules (fig. 6/10) should be broadcast on television and appear in the newspapers at the beginning of the winter ski season, and be explained to children and young people by their parents and teachers. Ski instructors should provide compulsory courses on the rules for all their pupils, just as car drivers are instructed in the rules of behavior on the road.

In the USA, one ski school teaches ski safety in its beginner's classes. No serious injury to the class members has occurred during this study period [23].

(1) Consideration for others – Every skier must always behave in such a way that he does not endanger or harm someone else.

(2) Control of speed and manner of skiing – Every skier must adapt his speed and manner of skiing to his proficiency and to the prevailing slope and weather conditions.

(3) Choice of ski track – The skier coming from behind must choose his track in such a way so as not to endanger the person skiing ahead of him.

(4) Passing – May be done above or below, on the right or the left, but always with enough distance to allow the skier being passed sufficient room for all his movements.

(5) Responsibilities of skiers lower down and crossing – Every skier who is about to enter a descent slope or wants to cross a slope (traverse) must first look up and down and around to make sure that he may do so without any danger to himself and others. The same is true after each stop.

(6) Stopping on descent slope – Every skier must avoid stopping at narrow or view-obstructing spots on a descent slope. A skier who falls must try to leave such spots as promptly as possible.

(7) Climbing – A climbing skier may only use the side of a descent slope; he must also leave the slope if visibility is poor. This also applies to a person descending on foot.

(8) Obeying signs – Every skier must obey all signs posted on the ski slopes.

(9) Behavior in case of accidents – In case of an accident everybody is obliged to render assistance.

(10) Identification obligation in case of accidents – Everyone, whether witness or involved, must identify himself when an accident occurs.

Discussion

It is clear that indirect preventive measures are not easy especially for children and young skiers [41, 44]. Nevertheless, they may prevent firstly direct or indirect head injuries, and secondly many other injuries, such as fracture of the upper or lower leg.

Children must be advised by their parents, and adults must decide for themselves what is safe. There are no enforceable rules like when driving a car, for example, nor are there speed limitations or traffic lanes on the slopes. Coordination and cooperation by all are necessary for the known indirect preventive measures to be applied. It should be the responsibility of television, newspapers, insurance companies and tourist information centers to publicise the safety rules and methods of accident prevention, and, especially for children, the family and educational facilities could help too.

Skiing is a free sport, yet the enforcement of safety regulations by the State may nevertheless be required, because, being the national sport here in Switzerland, it now causes too many accidents leading to serious personal family and social consequences.

Direct Preventive Measures: The Safety Helmet

As I have mentioned before, the so-called indirect factors alone are not sufficient to prevent accidents, particularly head injuries.

Direct accident prevention measures are also required, and one which is simple and very sensible is to wear a 'helmet' (fig. 6/8, 6/26).

In many types of sport, such as ice hockey, hang gliding, canoeing, parachute jumping, rock climbing, American football, the wearing of this simple, direct head protection is a matter of course.

Thus, car racing and downhill ski racing without a helmet are unjustifiable, considering that it is compulsory to wear a helmet in ice hockey games and motorcycle races. Virtually no head injuries occur in cross-country skiing because of the very low speed involved. I have never yet had to treat a patient for head injuries incurred during cross-country skiing.

Far be it from me to discourage skiers from taking part in this fascinating sport, but I do strongly urge that a safety helmet be worn as the only feasible and sensible direct measure to prevent injury to the head and brain, and even to the neck (see fig. 6/23–25).

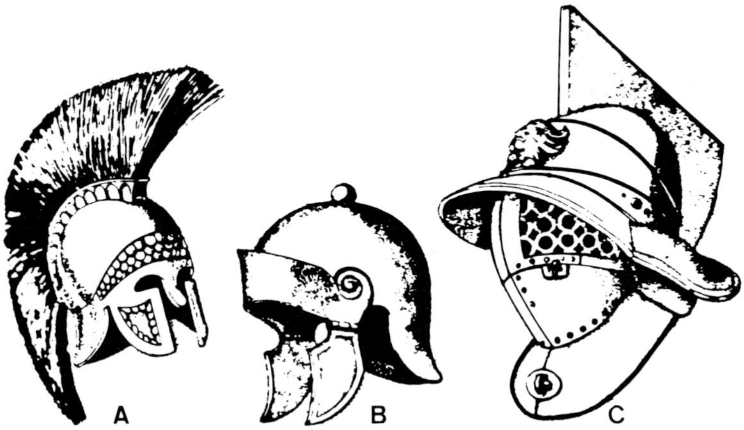

Fig. 6/11. **A** Greek warrior of about 500 BC. **B** Roman legionary of the first century AD. **C** Roman gladiator of the second century AD.

History

The helmet covering and protecting the head is one of the oldest items of armour.

Although there were earlier protective head coverings, most studies of helmets start from those worn in ancient Greece and Rome (fig. 6/11). Helmets are usually thought of today as items of military equipment – for soldiers, sailors or airmen [12].

New and modified types are worn by firemen, miners, construction workers, racing drivers and others engaged in hazardous occupations, as well as in many kinds of sport.

Helmets were initially made of hard leather and bronze. On some of these types the neck and the ears were protected, and some even had a rudimentary visor. In northern and western Europe the first helmets were made of leather reinforced with bronze or iron straps. Gradually, the amount of metal increased until entire helmets of iron were fashioned, still following the same straps.

About the year 1000, a bar projecting downward from the front rim, called a nasal, was added to protect the nose. The desire for still further protection led to the development of the helm, or heaume, at about 1200. At first, almost a straight, flat-topped cylinder, they then gradually assumed rounded contours that would cause blows to glace off, and they were extended downward to protect the neck. Shortly after 1300, a movable visor was added to cover the face.

About the year 1400, the great bascinet appeared. The 15th century, which witnessed the appearance of the bascinet, also brought forth three other types of helmets, all deriving from the same simple bascinet. The real advance in helmet design, however, came with the armet, and later the close helmet. The armet and close helmet changed all that. By hingeing the cheek pieces, as on the armet, or pivoting them, as on the close helmet, armourers produced a helmet that could fit tightly under the chin and base of the skull. This design fully protected the neck but made it possible for a blow to dislodge the helmet in battle.

The evolution of the armet began shortly after 1400 and the close helmet appeared about 1500. Both were truly closed helmets and continued in use as long as full helmets were worn. About 1550, however, two new types, the morion and the cabasset, became popular. The cabasset had a pointed, keeled bowl or crown and a narrow brim. The morion had a round bowl with a high comb and a crescent-shaped brim rising to points at the front and back. They were worn by nearly all infantry and by ceremonial guards and by almost everyone who desired a light helmet. Their period of popularity lasted until about 1650, though the Papal Swiss guard continues to wear them in the 20th century.

During the 16th century there also appeared a very versatile helmet known as a burgonet.

In the 17th century, a particular form of a burgonet with a neck defence of overlapping plates became popular, and it was called a lobster-tail burgonet because of the supposed resemblance to the plates of a lobster's abdomen or tail. Light horsemen were particularly fond of the burgonet and it became almost standard equipment for them throughout Europe until near the end of the 17th century.

With the decline of the full helmet late in the 17th century, attention was focused on the light metal skullcap that could be worn under the regular cloth hat. Such caps became standard for dragoons, heavy cavalry and for many officers, and were worn throughout the next century.

Some infantry officers wore them as late as World War I. In 1750, it became the custom to equip the newly developed light cavalry with helmets of hard leather in England, France and other European nations.

During the 19th century, leather, brass and even steel helmets became fashionable for various types of cavalry. Although some infantry regiments, notably those of Germany, wore leather helmets bound with metal, the steel helmet did not reappear as a regulation item of equipment until the time of World War I.

The French first adopted the helmet as standard in 1914, the British in 1915, followed quickly by the Germans and then by the rest of Europe and the United States. All were designed with glancing surfaces so that a bullet or shell fragment would bounce off without imparting its full impact.

During World War II, after continued research by armour specialists, several new models were brought forth – issued for soldiers, sailors and airmen.

After World War II synthetic products were developed and plastic helmets appeared made of materials such as polyester, polyamide, polyethylene, polycarbonate and fibreglass (resin reinforced with glass fibre). These plastic helmets were brought into sporting, traffic, domestic, professional and industrial fields mostly. Both in health and recreation, modern human life has become more dangerous mainly due to scientific development. There is also more chance of head accidents occurring.

New thermoplastic materials (e.g. high impact polyamide) have proved to be better functionally, i.e., resistant to heat, cold and impact forces. They are of remarkably low density, resistant to numerous solvents and alcaly, unaffected by petrol oils, and easy to process.

The characteristics of formation of the plastic helmets differ, serving special purposes also in sport performance. Technical advance, medical experience and research work must collaborate in making a better and optimal version.

Preventive Functions

The helmet must be able to protect against injury in case of accident. The application of kinetic force to the head causes various types of injuries which can be differentiated into 4 types as follows:

(1) Penetrating injury: A small-area object (fig. 4/10) with, for instance, a point or a sharp edge, penetrates the skull, leading to a depressed fracture which is one typical kind of skiing injury. This often happens on collision with various obstacles, causing an open or closed depressed fracture with or without brain lesions. The curved, hard, glancing surface of the outer shell of the helmet protects the head against penetrating injuries (fig. 6/12), by deflecting most of the kinetic energy.

6/12 6/13

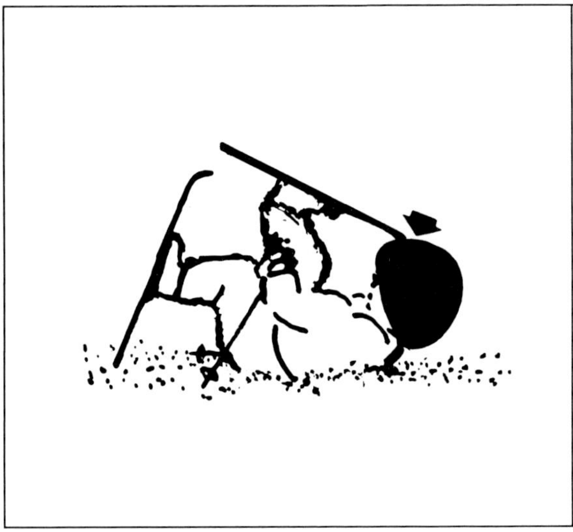

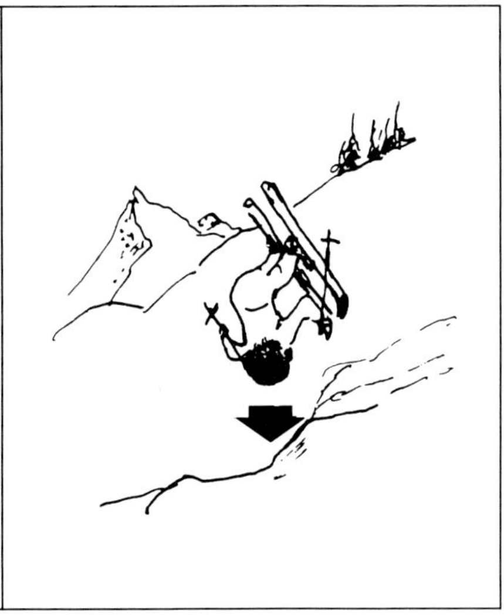

Fig. 6/12. Helmet prevents piercing injury by ski tip (outer shell of helmet provides protection).

Fig. 6/13. Hitting the hard slope at high speed caused a deceleration injury.

(2) Deceleration injury: Application of force over a large area (fig. 4/7) will mostly cause brain damage: the so-called retardation injury. This usually occurs in a fall on icy or hard ski slopes. Furthermore, skiing at high speed and hitting the slope can cause a closed brain injury, as in the case No. 7 of a young skier where an acute contusion hematoma led to his death (fig. 6/13). The soft cushioned inner shell of the helmet (see fig. 6/20) usually prevents deceleration injury to the head.

(3) Pressure injury: This type of head injury does not occur in skiing accidents. These injuries mainly happen in American football and usually lead to serious brain damage, such as an acute brain contusion hematoma that may be fatal [17, 60]. The energy of impact over a large area is transmitted to the brain, with or without an initial linear skull fracture, and then hitting the opposite side of the head causes reflection of the deceleration energies, which are transmitted to the brain again (fig. 6/14).

(4) Lacerations (scalp injury): This type of injury happens in all sorts of ski accidents, with or without craniocerebral injuries.

Indirect protection factors should also be mentioned. The helmet protects against wind, sunshine, snowfall, rain, dirt and especially cold while skiing (fig. 6/15).

6/14

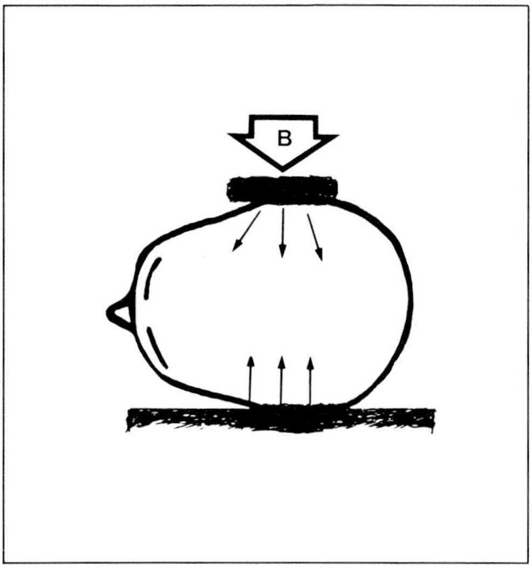

6/15

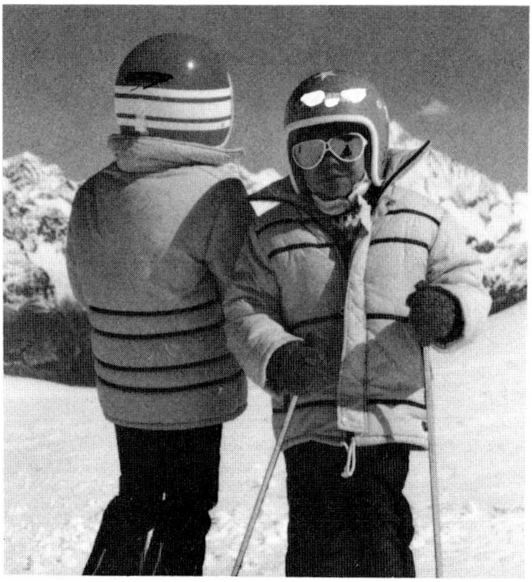

Fig. 6/14. A force of deceleration over a large area causes injury to the brain, and reflection of the same energies to the opposite side of the brain by a fixed object, such as the ground or a wall. B = Direction of impact.

Fig. 6/15. Helmet is better protection against cold than is a cap.

Clinical Observation

The skier is pilot and vehicle all in one (according to the television commentators last skiing season). Lacking a tachometer, he is unable to measure his speed objectively and cannot control it when racing at more than 140 km/h (the speed limit for cars on highways is 120 km/h) down unsafe slopes.

Skiing is a relaxation and recreation, but it also entails hazards to life and limb, since (unlike in car accidents) all forces are absorbed by the body. To date I have seen five skiing accidents to children/young people where each wore a safety helmet. Thanks to this helmet no dangerous head injuries occurred, although judging from the speed, force of impact and marks on the helmet this would have been expected.

One such case is that of a 16-year-old boy (case 37) who fell during downhill training on the open slope. His speed at the time of his fall was about 80 km/h. He was wearing a safety helmet (fig. 6/16A, B), but his head hit the hard ski slope and he suffered a head injury. Most of the force was deflected by the helmet. He had a mild brain contusion and left brachial nerve contusion which were treated conservatively. Without the helmet the

A 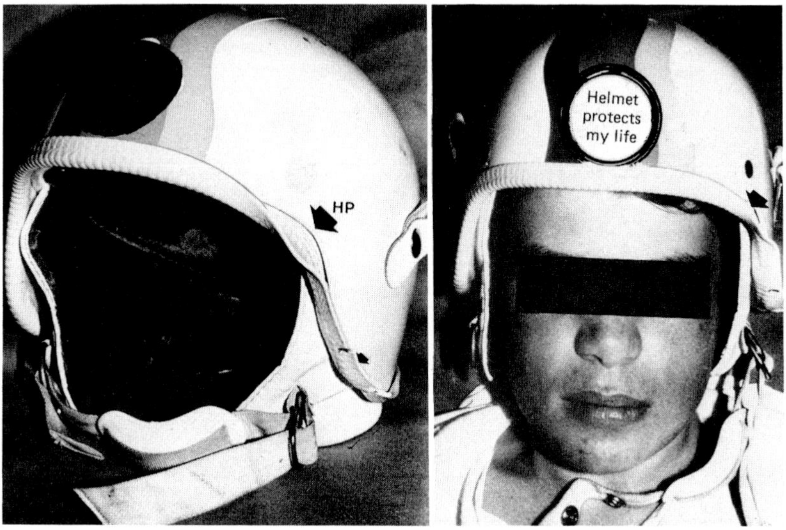 B

Fig. 6/16. A Case 37. Helmet damaged in the left temporal region (HP). HP = Point of impact. **B** Safety helmet saved his life.

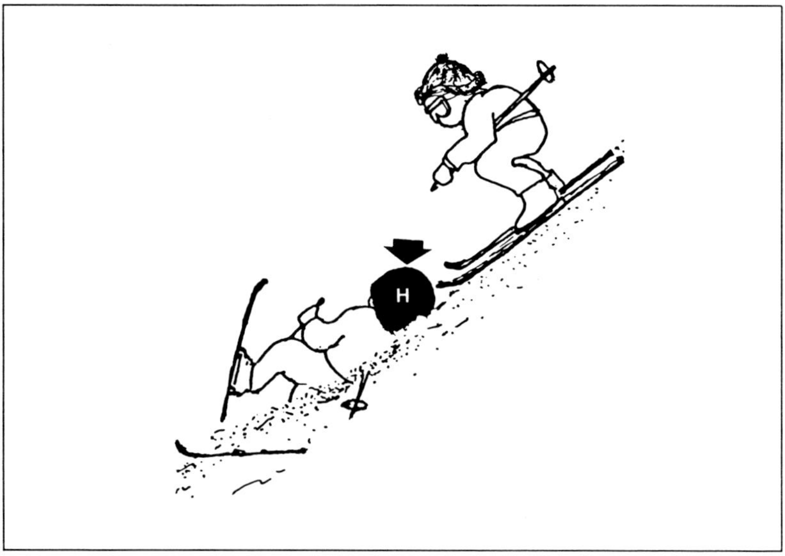

Fig. 6/17. If this injured skier had worn a helmet, the fatal head injury would most likely have been prevented. H = Safety helmet.

Table 6/I. Fatal cases (1975–1982)

Patient No.	Date	Age/sex	Cause of accident
1	Feb. 1975	22/F	collided with another skier
2	April 1976	14/M	crashed against obstacle
3	April 1979	19/M	fell and slid
4	Feb. 1979	23/M	fell from ski-lift
5	Feb. 1979	9/M	slipped and fell
6	Jan. 1980	11/F	another skier collided
7	Feb. 1980	18/M	fell after jump
8	Feb. 1980	22/M	collided with another skier
9	Feb. 1980	24/M	fell after jump
10	Feb. 1980	44/F	tumbled over on mountain
11	Mar. 1980	47/M	collided wih another skier
12	Dec. 1980	18/M	fell and slid
13	Mar. 1981	27/F	collided with another skier
14	April 1981	40/M	slid off
15	Dec. 1982	28/M	collided with obstacle
16	Dec. 1982	30/M	slid off

full force would have been exerted on the head and then the young skier would have suffered a serious head injury.

Severe head injuries may lead to a permanent handicap and this often results in serious family and social problems. Admissions to hospital and surgical procedures, absence from school, memory deterioration, post-traumatic syndromes such as headaches, dizziness and convulsive seizures could be reduced considerably, to say nothing of the known mortality in our region alone every year.

I have dealt with many tragic skiing accident cases where the outcome was fatal. Seven happened in the year 1980, and most involved children and young skiers (table 6/I) [42].

Two-thirds of the fatal head injuries were the fault of those injured (deviation from slope, collision with an obstacle, etc.).

As some other authors have also pointed out, these accidents can be attributed to insufficient physical training, and uncontrolled, fast and careless skiing. This type of accident seems to happen predominantly to boys and young men.

One-third of these tragic head injuries were not the fault of those injured. They generally affected slower and careful skiers involved in collisions on an open slope with fast skiers (fig. 6/17) [41].

6/18
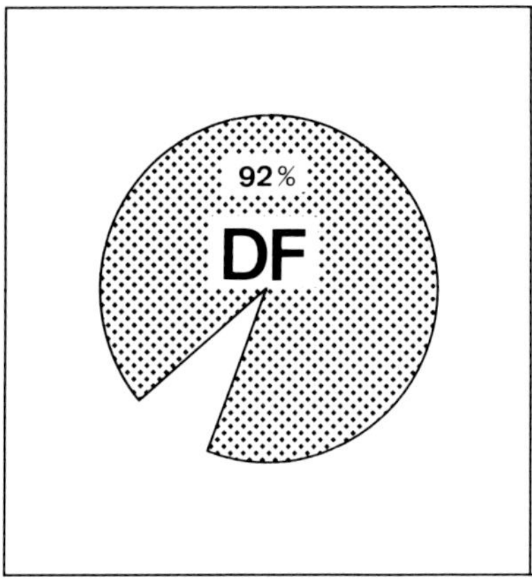

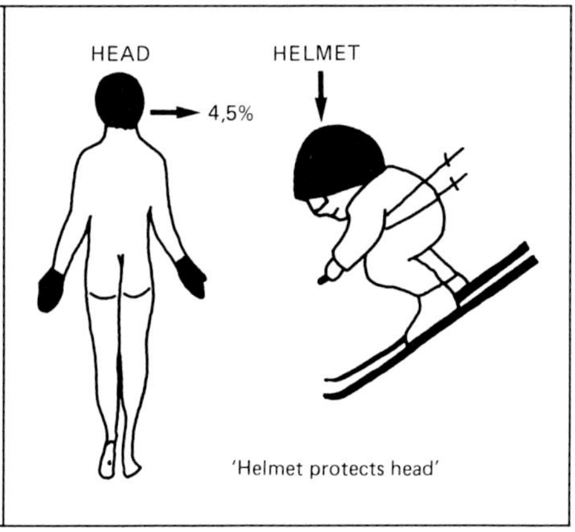

6/19

Fig. 6/18. 92% depressed fractures of children/young skiers. DF = Depressed skull fracture.

Fig. 6/19. The head protected by a helmet is 4.5% of the body surface area, equivalent to two gloved hands.

As I have mentioned many times elsewhere, head injuries with depressed skull fractures and possibly with brain damage/haemorrhage occur very often (the classical type of head injuries) to children and young skiers (about 92%) (fig. 6/18) [44]. These depressed fractures required several operations including artificial covering of the damage (fig. 3/13) This is the great problem with these injuries, which could certainly be prevented by wearing a safety helmet.

Skiing involves downward movement on the oblique plane of a mountain-side (fig. 4/4), and a fronto-frontal collision of heads with another downhill skier is normally impossible, unlike car accidents. However, direct frontal collisions of the head with obstacles (trees, rock, ski-lift pylon, electric pylon, brick wall, ski stands, etc.) are among the most frequent causes of accidents, as has been pointed out previously.

Ideal Protection

By wearing a saftey helmet, i.e. by protecting just 4.5% of body surface area (equal to the area of two gloved hands), it is possible to prevent severe head injuries in a simple, reliable and economical manner (fig. 6/19).

All types of head injuries in skiing accidents could be prevented by a proper safety helmet.

6/20 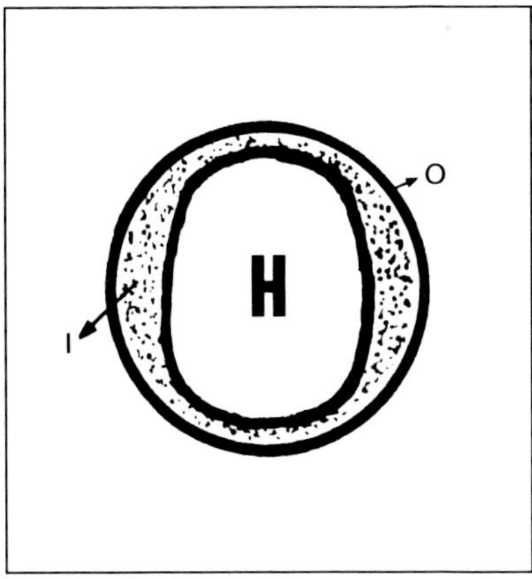

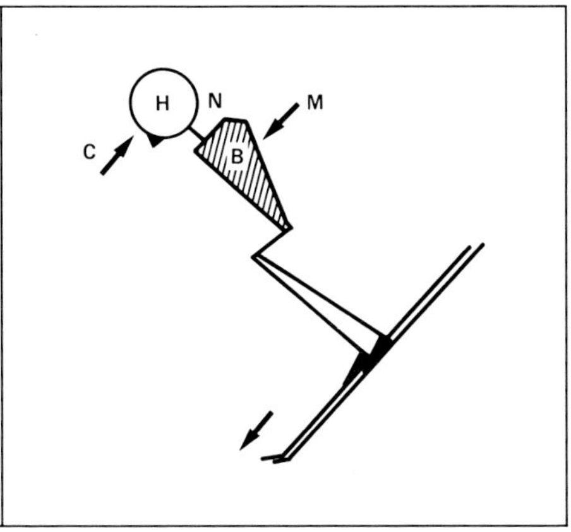 6/21

Fig. 6/20. Horizontal section throught a safety helmet. H = Head; O = curved outer shell; I = cushioned inner shell.

Fig. 6/21. Illustration of cervical injury. H = Head; N = neck; B = body; C = collision; M = direction of motion.

The curved and smooth outer shell (fig. 6/20, O) very reliably prevents penetating injuries, and it will partly deflect the impinging object and thus the energy of impact. When a head injury occurs, the direction of application of force and the particlar region of the skull affected are of considerable importance. As the illustration indicates, a circular cross-section is important, since this is particularly effective for reducing temporoparietal injuries which mostly result in serious injuries in skiing accidents. This curved helmet shell can actually deflect the energy of impact of most objects, in contrast to a flat surface, and thus prevents injuries (fig. 4/26).

The remaining energy of impact, and this also applies to collision with blunt objects, will be considerably neutralised by the soft-cushioned inner shell of the helmet, so that the force transmitted to the head, and particularly to the brain, which gives rise to deceleration injuries, is very much reduced.

Additional Advantages

The energy of frontal collision causes decerebrate damage to the brain and cervical spine injuries if the force is applied over a large area (without an open skull fracture, especially depressed fracture) (fig. 6/21).

Cervical spine injuries (isolated or combined) from skiing accidents are not uncommon [48].

Table 6/II. Age and sex relations

Age, years	Male	Female	Total
10–17	6	1	7
18–30	3	1	4
31–40	–	2	2
Over 41	4	1	5
Total	13	5	18

Table 6/III. Causes of the accidents, lesions to and treatment of the cervical spine

Patient No.	Age/sex	Cause	Lesion	Treatment	Year
1	42/M (FRG)	fall	FD/C6-7+CC	CD (Op)	1978
2	17/M (FRG)	fall	FD/C4-5+CC	Tr	1978
3	15/M	fall	FD/C5-6+CC	Tr	1979
4[1]	36/M	collision	FD/C4-5+CC	CD (Op)	1979
5	10/M	funicular	FD/C3-4	Co	1979
6	55/M (France)	fall	FD/C6-7+CC	Tr	1980
7	17/M	fall	FD/C4-5	Co	1980
8	45/F	fall	FD/C5-6+CC	Co	1980
9	35/F	fall	FD/C5-6+CC	CD (Op)	1980
10	8/F	fall	FD/C2-3	Co	1980
11	28/F (FRG)	collision	FD/C2-3+CC	Death	1981
12	37/F	fall	FD/C4-5+CC	Co	1982
13	30/M	fall	FD/C4-5+CC	Co	1982
14	57/M (NL)	fall	FD/C5-6	Tr	1982
15[2]	16/M	collision	FD/C4-5+CC	CD (Op)	1983
16	27/M	aerial maneuver	FD/C1-2	Co	1983
17	15/M	aerial maneuver	FD/C2-3+CC	Co	1983
18	19/M (FRG)	fall	FD/C6-7	Tr	1983

FD = Fracture-dislocation; CC = cerebral contusion; CD (Op) = Cloward operation; Tr = transportation; Co = conservative treatment.

[1] Case 38.

[2] Case 39.

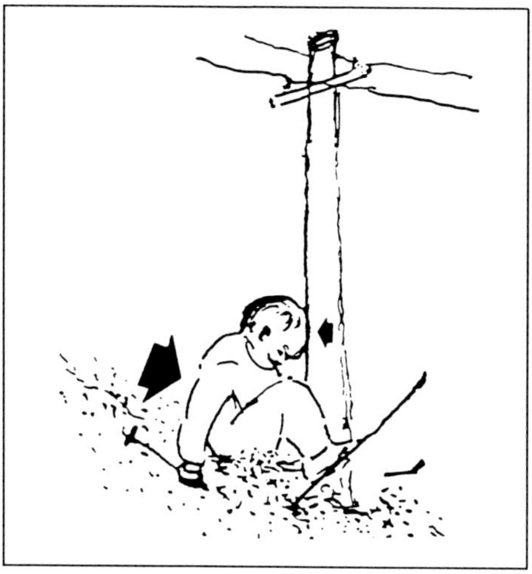

Fig. 6/22. Violent collision with telegraph pole, causing severe cervical fracture-dislocation and head injury.

A downhill skier's body is moving forward, of course. In a collision, the head usually makes first contact, causing direct injury, then the flexible and relatively weak cervical region receives indirect rebound blows anterior-posteriorly. A fracture-dislocation of the cervical spine may occasionally be the result of the violent blow.

I have described 18 patients (in a retrospective study) with cervical spine injury [48]. 4 patients were treated surgically for instability. 12 patients (67%) also had head injuries, of whom 2 patients underwent surgery.

Between 1978 and 1983 (5 years) 18 patients with cervical spine injuries were treated (table 6/II). The incidence for males was high, 13 cases (72%), and 7 patients (40%) were below 17 years of age. 12 patients suffered slight to severe head injuries, and 1 patient died (table 6/III, patient No. 11) from complete fracture-dislocation of C2-C3 with severe cerebral contusion caused by collision with another skier where ski slopes crossed.

Two examples of accidents resulting in cervical spine injury (cases 38 and 39) are now presented.

Case 38; a 36-year-old male, is in charge of rescues at the slope complex at Flims. During an inspection trip in January 1979, he collided with a telegraph pole (fig. 6/22), hitting his head violently. According to his statement he was unconscious for more than an hour.

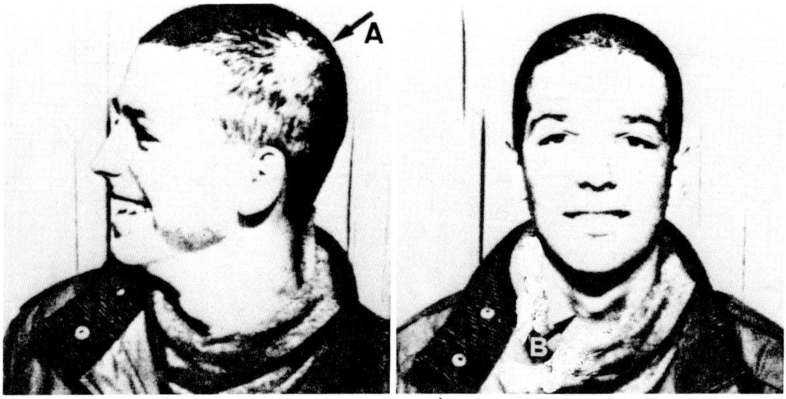

A B

Fig. 6/23. Healthy patient after third operation. **A** After skull operation. **B** After cervical spine operation.

He was able to call for help using his own radio, and was transported by sled to the valley and by helicopter to our neurosurgical department where he complained of severe pain in the cervical region and the head. Cervical spine X-ray revealed a fracture-dislocation C5/6. After dressing the large laceration wound on the head, a head/skeletal tongs traction was applied. The patient subsequently recuperated rather well and the neurological signs slowly disappeared. After reduction of the fracture-dislocation, surgery was performed (fig. 3/59). Postoperative recovery was completely without complications. The patient could be sent home in good general condition 3 weeks later, without any neurological deficits.

Case 39, a 16-year-old male, fell and collided with stone objects at the side of the skiing slope. He was conscious on admission. Skull X-rays showed a left parietal open depressed fracture and dislocation C4 and C5 with stretching of the spine. He underwent immediate surgery (head and spine). 3 weeks later the patient was sent home in good general condition. The left parietal skull defect was treated 3 months later by Palacos cranioplasty (fig. 6/23).

The position of the skier's head is as typical as the boxer's head position, that is, the head is forward and the shoulders are raised (crouched posture (fig. 4/4b.).

In this position, it is certain that a rear extension to the safety helmet (fig. 6/24) would provide additional protection against cervical spine injury (fig. 6/25).

6/24
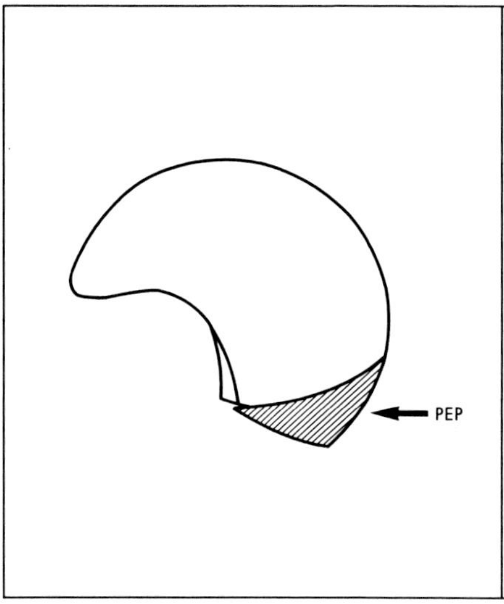

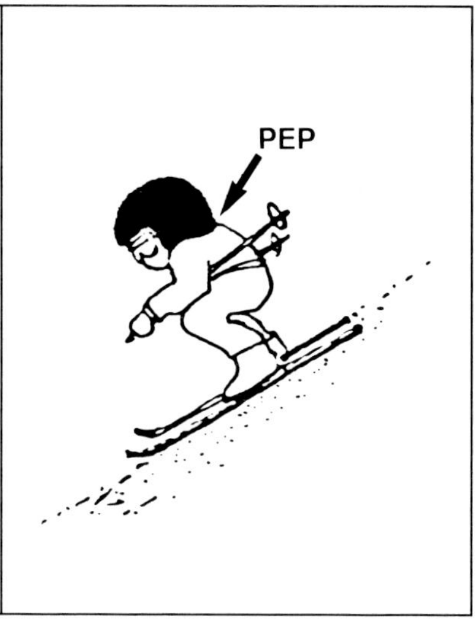

6/25

Fig. 6/24. Posterior extended part (PEP) protects against cervical spine injuries.
Fig. 6/25. Modern helmet protects against head and neck injuries.

Discussion

Wearing a safety helmet instead of a woollen cap can reduce head injuries and, in particular, prevent the tragic fatalities [33, 39, 40–42, 44, 46–48].

We all know that it is necessary to provide children and young people with optimal life protection [44]. For instance, the minimum age for driving a car is 18 years, and for boxing it is 14 years.

Skiers increasingly imitate their idols in the ski race circuit, which itself is becoming more dangerous each year. Stimulated by their example, skiing becomes faster and more reckless, and this on slopes with ever greater traffic congestion!

I have detailed the many ways accidents can occur and the head injuries which result: falls on icy slopes, and collision with various obstacles, including the tips of one's own skis. Just being careful is not sufficient, because collisions with other slope users are frequent.

Children and young skiers are often victims of accidents causing injuries to the skull and brain, and there is a trend for these to increase. For participants in ski races (as for similarly endangered motorcyclists in street

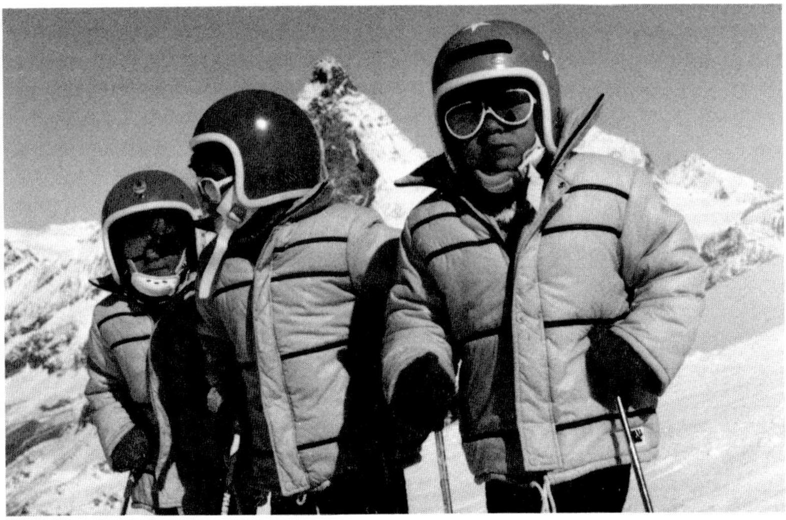

Fig. 6/26. Smart heads protect themselves and a helmet saves life.

traffic) the safety helmet has long been part of the standard equipment. We are not aware of a single racing skier suffering even slight head injuries in the last few years, and this is quite remarkable in view of the many spectacular falls and the, sometimes serious, injuries to other parts of the body.

Wearing a safety helmet is very advisable not only for children but for adults as well. A very tragic fatal head injury of an adult in a skiing accident (caused by himself) has been described. I had never before seen such a severe head injury (cases 19 and 20). Because of the growing number of skiers and the parallel increase in head injuries, simple, direct preventive measures are necessary.

The head injuries described here could certainly have been avoided, or at least reduced, had the patient worn a helmet (fig. 4/26). This case represents the most serious head injury of any skier I have seen so far at our hospital. Preventive medicine is the most up-to-date medicine, particularly for head injuries, because little progress in the therapy of these can be achieved. Education to prevent head injuries from skiing is much more important than treatment, because the former promises more success.

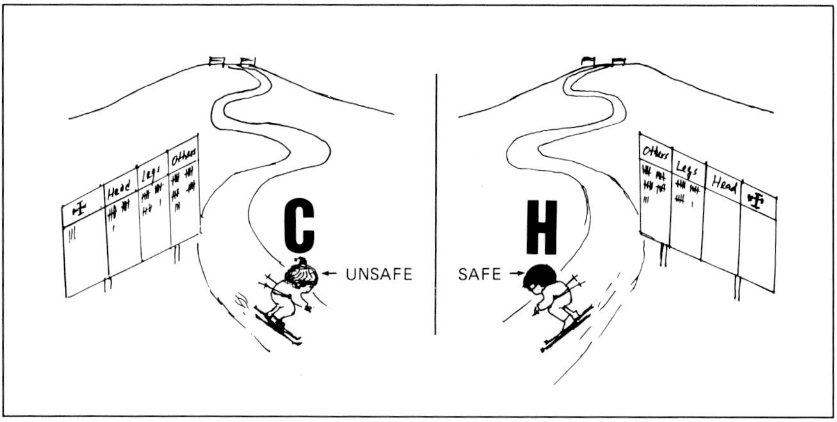

Fig. 6/27. Safe with helmet – no head injury or death (H). Unsafe without helmet – head injuries and even some fatal accidents (C). H = Helmet; C = cap.

Similar to the compulsory wearing of helmets by motor cyclists, it is essential in skiing for the safety helmet to replace the woollen cap for both adults and children (fig. 6/27). At the beginning of every skiing season, the importance of the safety helmet must be emphasised. This represents a simple, inexpensive and effecitve way of preventing head injuries while skiing.

7 History of Skiing as a Sport

It is not known for sure who the first skiers were nor who invented the ski. Maybe research will provide definite answers in the future. What is known today is that the ski was already used as a means of travel far back in ancient times. The Japanese, Chinese, Persians, Caucasians as well as the Indians in Alaska used snowshoes, and in the far north, in Siberia and in the Scandinavian countries, the ski has been in use for thousands of years, because in those endless, almost flat snow deserts it represented the most natural means of getting around.

The oldest figurative exhibition of skiing is a rock-drawing discovered in Norway, dating back to the Stone Age in the opinion of the experts, and in a Nordic museum a ski alleged to be 2,500 years old is displayed [35].

The Greek historian *Xenophon,* around 400 BC, reports observing that the mountain-people in Armenia tied sackcloth around the hoofs of their horses, to prevent them from sinking into the snow deeply. *Strabo,* at a later date, describes that round discs were used by the Armenians instead of sackcloth. Those may have been the first snow-shoes of a type used until recent times for crossing mountains in the winter time.

In the Far East the snowshoe has been known for a long time too. In historical annals of the Tang dynasty which ruled from 618 until 907 AD, we find the following sentence about the Kirghese, for instance: 'When snow has fallen, they hunt their animals on wooden horses.' For that reason they were also called the 'Wooden-horse Turks'. *Arianos* reports about a march by Roman legions across Armenian snowfields during one of the military campaigns of the Roman emperor *Ulpius Trajanus* (98–117 AD).

Another historian tells us that the Byzantine emperor *Leo* and 50 of his men crossed the Caucasian mountains on skis in the year 710 AD. About the people of Asia Minor it is reported in 852 AD that they drove down mountain slopes on snowshoes that were fastened to their feet. In an account from the year 1307 about a Mongol clan of the Baykal-Lake region we read: 'As there is a lot of snow in their land they busily hunt on the snow in winter. For this purpose they made wooden boards, fastened them to

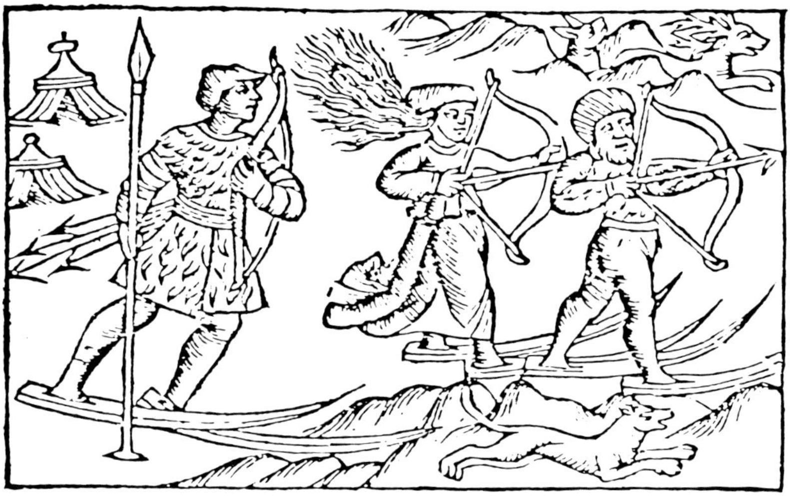

Fig. 7/1. Lapps skiing [from Olaus Magnus: Historia de gentibus septentrionalibus, Roma 1535, German edition (Geschichte der mitternächtlichen Völker), Basel 1967].

their feet with straps, and in that manner hunted across the steppes and plains, uphill and downhill.'

A bit more is known about the use of snowshoes and skis by the Nordic people. For the Lapps, for instance, the ski represented the only means to follow their reindeerherds and keep them together. Even bears were hunted on skis, since the Lapps did all their hunting on these wooden gliding implements. The people of ancient times knew for instance that the Lapps and the Finns were called 'Skridfinns' by the Normans – 'skrid' means sliding or gliding; and because the Finns were very skilful in the use of their wooden skis they were named 'Skridfinns'. In any case, the 'Königsspiegel' (Royal Mirror) of the year 1250 reports that some of the male hunters were so proficient of their gliding implements that they could kill nine and more reindeer with their spears while in motion.

As to the question of where the ski was invented ... it is generally assumed that it was in Norway. Yet, the Swedish Roman Catholic bishop *Olaus Magnus* pointed to another origin. During the reformation he was banned from Uppsala in the year 1535, and while exiled in Rome he wrote a 'Geschichte der mitternächtlichen Völker' (History of the midnight people). In this book the Lapps are praised as good skiers (fig. 7/1) [38].

Olaus Magnus, who is also well known as a cartographer, gives an accurate description of the ski models, ski sticks and furskin coverings

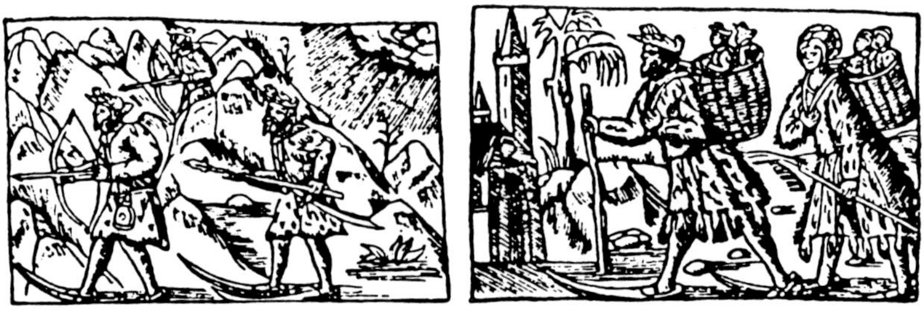

Fig. 7/2. Hunting and travelling 'Skridfinns' [from the Northern Chronicle of Olaus Magnus, 1555].

commonly used in those days. He also gave us the first information in 1555 about competitive ski sport events [35]. Skiing was considered a chivalrous sport in Scandinavia, and is described as such in the 'Edda' as well as in the 'Wielandsaga'. Legend has it that the first settlers of Norway came on skis.

Nansen refers to this in his work 'Nebelheim' (Fog-home) and quotes the following paragraph from the 'Historia Norwegiae': 'The Finns are excellent hunters, they roam around constantly, living in huts made of skins [15]. These huts they carry on their shoulders, they fasten smooth wooden pieces to their feet (actually planks, sticks), which they call Ondrer, and while the wives and children move across the steep mountains in deep snow, they themselves scurry around faster than a bird.' There are still some pictures in existence today which show that even the women of the Skridfinns participated in the hunting and wore snowshoes (fig. 7/2).

In the third chapter of the first book of the 'Skridfinns' (Lapps), we read: 'Instead of shoes the inhabitants of this land wear smooth woods, pointed in the front ... they tie them to the feet, hold a stick in the hand with which to lead, and as it pleases them, backward, forward, sideways, downward or upward, with amazing speed they go and slide, over the tops of snow-mountains.'

From these few references it is evident that the ski in its early form – which of course had little in common with the skiing equipment of today, yet must be considered the forerunner of it – played an important role as a means of travel and in the struggle for existence. It is not surprising, therefore, that it was also utilized in war in the old days. We have proof that in March of the year 1200, during the battle of Isen near Oslo, the ski was definitely used, and it is considered likely that the Swedes introduced the ski into central Europe during the 30-year war; though it sank into oblivion again later on [15]. Others point out that ski remnants were dug up from the moors of northern Europe, but never found in those of Siberia. Is this any proof, though? Most likely, the people there simply never bothered to dig for ski remnants in their swamps and moors.

Some believe that the ski had its origin somewhere in central Siberia, around the region of the Baykal Lake and the Sajan-Altai mountains, and that it spread from there to the north, east and west, similar to the way described by Nansen to indicate ski names on his map. However, because the ski is so very old, nobody really has been able to pin the honour of fatherhood on any specific people up to now. The ski as a means of travel was invented some 2,000 years ago, it became a first class sporting gadget in later years. Only recently has it developed again into a travelling device in some areas: in northern Europe, in Alaska, in Russia, and in every Swiss mountain village moving around in the winter time is now done on skis. Pupils and teachers go to school on their woods, even the minister puts on his beloved skis to get to his church or to perform his other duties in the Alpine village. Thus, the circle has been closed.

Aren't the Lapps the inventors of the ski then? The Finnish national poem 'Kalewala', referring to the Lapps as the fathers of the ski, seems to support this theory also. Yet, when one discovers that the ski was known in ancient times not only in Sweden, Norway, Finland and Lappland, but also in Russia, far into Siberia, one must assume that the use of the ski actually spread from the Far West to the Far East of the Euro-Asian continent. To bear this out, some authors claim that the ski was highly developed in the west, but quite primitive in the east. However this is not really true: in fact, the East-Siberian ski is highly sophisticated.

In Russian-Poland the ski apparently came into use during the 17th century [62]. In the book 'In honour of the Duchy Crain (Zur Ehre des Herzogtums Crain), which appeared in Laibach in 1689, we find a paragraph with the peculiar title: 'About strange crossing of snow-mountains.' As an oddity, so to speak, it is described there that Crainish peasants crossed the mountains on snow-hoops and also walked across snow. The author Baron *von Valvasor* writes about skiers: 'No mountain is too steep, nor covered too much with large trees, to prevent them from driving downhill in that manner, for they twist their descent like snakes when some obstacles block the way, be it a tree or a large rock. But when the route is all clear and unobstructed, they glide down straight as an arrow.' Judging from these descriptions the Crainish peasants must have developed a considerable skiing technique, keeping in mind their primitive gliding woods and bindings; for these people obviously knew nothing yet of Splittkein-ski, of Kandahar-binding and diagonal pull, of Rominger-Blue edge or Jack-Ettinger edge. The Christiania or the Telemark were not known to them either, nor the ski-school courses by Christian Rubi. For all of these are achievements of our present time, after all.

Still, competitive ski sport events did take place even in the Middle Ages. One can visualize the Finns and Lapps, the Kirghese and others, conducting popular games using skis. For just as hunting on skis or fighting a battle on skis demanded skill, and just as the knights had games to demonstrate their skill, agility and strength, so were sporting events conducted using long woods. The first ski-run competition with prize distribution is said to have taken place in 1767 in Christiania. The story is told of a Norwegian hero named Trysil Knud, who could jump over 12 men, firing a rifle at the same time, and who showed various funny tricks while skiing; he won all the prizes at that time. How much skiing has progressed since then, particularly also with regard to ski sport competition, is well known to everybody.

In Central Europe the first ski appeared as early as the 16th century, but it was then used as a museum piece only, because nobody know what to do with it. It took a long time, however, until skiing as a sport became common in our region. The first skiers were laughed at and derided. The main reasons for this slow development here were the poor ski bindings and the inadequate skiing technique in use then, which were of particular disadvantage in the mountainous countries. Some daring feats by mountaineering and skiing pioneers helped finally to overcome the prejudices and for the Alpine skiers to be taken seriously. *Fridtjof Nansen's* crossing of Greenland on skis in 1890/1891, as well as a few crossings of the Alps in Switzerland, demonstrated beyond a doubt that the ski was indeed a useful tool for the mountains during the winter time [15].

Those pioneers in the usage of snowshoes, as these long woods were generally called until only a few decades ago were some young farmers from the Norwegian village of Telemarken, having invented the elegant swing hereafter known as the Telemark, which permitted a controlled downhill driving and fast braking even on steep slopes. Later, the Telemark was almost completely displaced by the flashy Christiania, so named after the Norwegian capital, now known as Oslo.

In our own country the first skis appeared in Davos and Arosa around 1880. Their owners did not quite know how to use them properly, however, and after a few unsuccessful attempts put them away again. In 1889, a Norwegian engineer named *Olaf Kielsberg*, who worked in Winterthur and was accustomed to the long woods from his homeland, hustled about on his skis all by himself, and 2 years later he climbed the 119 m high Bachtel hill in the Zurich Oberland on skis [35].

The honour of being the father of Swiss skiing belongs to *Christof Iselin* of Glarus, however, for his energetic and successful pioneering of the snowshoes. Spurred on by *Nansen's* book 'Auf Schneeschuhen durch Grönland' (On snowshoes across Greenland), the then only 22-year-old *Iselin* manufactured a pair of skis for himself and made some practice runs after dark, in order not to be seen and ridiculed. Though his experiments were not too encouraging, he persisted and even arranged for *Kielsberg* and another young Norwegian to visit Glarus in December of 1892, in order to demonstrate their skill. Animated by this success, *Iselin, Kielsberg* and two other youngsters crossed the Pragel pass on skis a few weeks later, thereby proving the suitability of these new snow-walking implements for the mountains also.

The Dutchman *Henry Hoek*, born in Davos, who 10 years later won the German skiing championship and afterwards wrote several books about skiing, undertook his first trial runs in the Schwarzwald area around the same time, on skis he had imported from Christiania for the sum of 20 Francs. The new sport found its first fans in other places too, in Pratigau, Chur, St. Gall, in the Urseren valley and in Thun. Starting from Biel, 2 young enthusiasts climbed the Chasseral mountain in 1893, and in Arosa Dr. *Staeubli* from Zurich managed to reach the 2,985 m high Aroser Rothorn. *Ulrich Wille*, later on a Major-General in the Swiss Army, as a young student trained on the Gurten near Bern on skis he had imported from Norway. It was the English, however, who were the first to really appreciate the beauty of our Alps in the winter time and who made our winter resorts popular.

The skier of today has no idea of the difficulties our snowshoe pioneers had to overcome, due to the primitive equipment and lack of proper skiing techniques. For instance, Russian rubber boots were considered well suited as footwear when worn over normal shoes; this according to a 1897 description by the progressively thinking *Iselin*.

In November 1893, the first Swiss ski club was founded by *Christof Iselin* and 12 other ski enthusiasts, with *Iselin* its president. He persuaded fellow-citizen *Melchior Jakober* to mass produce snowshoes, thus founding the first ski manufacturing plant in Central Europe.

8 References

1 Aang, E.: Verletzungsschutz beim Skisport. Sportarzt Sportmed. *8:* 209 (1972).

2 Alister, McR.; Brody, J.A.; Hammes, L.M.; Feltz, E.T.; Duncan, D.L.; Williams, M.L.: Epidemiology of ski injuries in the Anchorage area. Archs envirnm. Hlth *10:* 910 (1965).

3 Al Zain, T.; Siedschlag, W.D.; Szdzy, D.: Zur Diagnostik und Therapie der Schädelkalottenimpressionsfrakturen. Z. ärztl. Fortbild. *70:* 709–710 (1976).

4 Arthur, G.; Gross, B.S.: A new theory on the dynamics of brain concussion and brain injury. J. Neurosurg. *15:* 548–561 (1958).

5 Baumgartner, W.: Die Sicherheit der Skiabfahrt. Münch. med. Wschr. *102:* 2220 (1960).

6 Baumgartner, W.: Ergebnisse der konservativen Behandlung der Skifrakturen der Unterschenkel. Sportarzt *9:* 202 (1959).

7 Biener, K.; Fasler, S.: Sportunfälle, pp. 187–250 (Huber, Bern 1978).

8 Böhler, L.: Konservative oder operative Behandlung der Torsionsbrüche des Unterschenkels beim Skilaufen. Sportarzt *9:* 204 (1959).

9 Bucher, H.: Der Einfluss von Sicherheitsbindungen auf Skiunfälle. Starke Jugend, Freies Volk *12:* 270 (1966).

10 Campell, R., Sr.: Zur Häufung der Unterschenkelschaftsfrakturen bei jugendlichen Skifahrern. Sportarzt *2:* 34 (1963).

11 Earle, A.; Moritz, J.; Saviers, G.: Ski injuries. J. Am. med. Ass. *180:* 285 (1962).

12 Encyclopaedia Britannica: Helmet. *1973:* 335–336.

13 Ergebnisse Unfallerhebung Winter (1980–1983): Fachgruppe der Seilbahnen in der Sektion Verkehr der Tiroler Handelskammer.

14 Frutiger, A.; Oh, S.; Leutenegger, A.: Erfahrungen mit Hirndruckmessungen bei posthypoxischen und posttraumatischen Komata. Schweiz. med. Wschr. *112:* 1177–1179 (1982).

15 Georgi, A.: Aus der Geschichte des Skisportes. Davoser Rev. *18:* 72–75 (1942).

16 Gerschler, W.: Leistungszuwachs bei Training der Skiläufer, unter Berücksichtigung funktioneller Gesichtspunkte. Sportarzt *2:* 29 (1963).

17 Gosch, H.H.; Gooding, E.; Schneider, R.G.: Distortion and displacement of the brain in experimental head injuries. Surg. Forum *20:* 425–426 (1969).

18 Gurdjian, E.S.; Hodgson, V.R.; Thomas, L.M.; Patrick, L.M.: Significance of relative movements of scalp, skull and intracranial contents during impact injury of the head. J. Neurosurg. *29:* 70–72 (1968).

19 Gurdjian, E.S.: Impact head injury; mechanistic, clinical and preventive correlation, pp. 133–134 (Thomas, Detroit 1975).

20 Gutmann, J.; Weisbuch, J.; Wolf, M.: Ski injuries in 1972–73. J. Am. med. Ass. *10:* 1423 (1974).
21 Haddon, W.; Ellison, A.E.; Carvoll, R.E.: Ski injuries. Publ. Hlth Rep. *77:* 975 (1962).
22 Haid, B.: Tödliche Skiverletzungen im Einzugsgebiet der Chirurgischen Universitätsklinik Innsbruck von 1944–1954. Arch. orthop. Unfallchir. *47:* 105–114 (1955).
23 Harris, J.B.: Neurosurgical injuries in winter sports. The physician and sports medicine *11:* 111–122 (1983).
24 Hodgson, V.R.; Gurdjian, E.S.; Thomas, L.M.: Experimental skull deformation and brain displacement demonstrated by flash X-ray technique. J. Neurosurg. *25:* 549–552 (1966).
25 Hornof, Z.; Schmid, L.: Tödliche Skiunfälle – Letalität und Verhütung. Sportarzt *1:* 10–13 (1965).
26 Knoringer, P.: Sofortdeckung von Schädellücken bei offenen und geschlossenen Impressionsfrakturen des Hirnschädels mit Acrylharzkunststoff. Ein klinischer Vergleich zwischen Palos K und Refobacin-Palacos R. Neurochirurgia *22:* 18–23 (1979).
27 Kollar, W.A.F.: Neurochirurgische Indikationen bei Wintersportverletzungen. Wien. med. Wschr. *5:* 164 (1977).
28 Kraus, H.: Prevention and treatment of skiing injuries. J. Am. med. Ass. *169:* 1414 (1959).
29 Kröger, M.; Marin, K.: Zur Problematik der Versorgung offener Impressionsfrakturen der Schädelkalotte. Hefte-Unfallheilk. *138:* 113–116 (1979).
30 Lippert, H.; Käfer, H.: Dicken der Knochenschichten. Mschr. Unfallheilk. Invalidenw. *77:* 329–339 (1974).
31 Lugger, L.J.: Der Unfall des Freizeitläufers. Med. Sport *13:* 378 (1973).
32 McFadden, J.T.: Straticulate decompression of depressed skull fractures. Surgery Gynec. Obstet. *144:* 415–418 (1977).
33 Mang, W.R.; Mauer, P.C.: Der tödliche Skiunfall. Orthop. Klin. Techn. Univ. München *94:* 107 (1976).
34 Matter, P.: Skitraumatologie und Unfallprophylaxe. Schweiz. Z. Sozialvers. *1:* 10 (1976).
35 Müller, H.: Aus der Geschichte des Skifahrens. Bündner Kalender *114:* 19–23 (1955).
36 Nahum, A.M.; Gatts, J.D.; Gadd, C.W.; Danforth, I.: Impact tolerance of the skull and face. Proc. 12 Stapp Car Coach Conf., p. 26 (Society of Automotive Engineers, New York 1968).
37 Napravnik, C.: Kopfverletzungen beim Eishockey. Med. Sport *XII:* 45 (1976).
38 Obholzer, A.: Der Ski – Woher? Von wem? Schneehase *30:* 74–78 (1974).
39 Oh, S.: Die Verhütung der Kopfverletzungen beim Skifahren. Schweiz. Z. Sportmed. *4:* 157–167 (1979).
40 Oh, S.: Zunehmende Schädelhirn-Traumen durch Skiunfälle und ihre Prophylaxe. Schweiz. Ärztezschr. *62:* 132–135 (1981).
41 Oh, S.; Nisoli, M.: Schwere Kollisionskopfverletzungen beim Skifahren und ihre Prävention. Praxis *10:* 408–413 (1981).
42 Oh, S.; Balmer, K.; Tok, S.: Tödliche Schädelhirnverletzungen durch Skiunfälle und ihre Prophylaxe. Schweiz. Z. Sportmed. *4:* 137–141 (1981).

43 Oh, S.; Rüedi, M.: Depressed skull fracture in skiing and its experimental study. Int. J. Sports Med. *3:* 169–173 (1982).
44 Oh, S.; Schmid, U.D.: Kindliche Kopfverletzungen beim Skifahren und ihre optimale Prophylaxe. Z. Kinderchir. *38:* 66–72 (1982).
45 Oh, S.: Clinical and experimental morphological study of the depressed skull fracture. Acta neurochir. *68:* 111–121 (1983).
46 Oh, S.; Wieland, H.: Kopfverletzungen durch Skiliftunfälle und ihre Verhütung. Z. Magglingen *40:* 13–15 (1983).
47 Oh, S.; Schmid, U.D.: Schädel-Hirn-Verletzungen beim Skifahren und ihre Verhütung. Unfallheilkunde *86:* 226–229 (1983).
48 Oh, S.: Cervical injury in skiing. Int. J. Sports Med. *5:* 208–281 (1984).
49 Oh, S.: Experimental morphological study of the depressed skull fracture. Experimental models. Neurochirurgia *2:* 111–114 (1984).
50 Patscheider, H.: Todesfälle beim Wintersport. Wien med. Wschr. *41:* 669–672 (1961).
51 Pidermann, G.: Sicherheit im Skisport. Wer ist der Tausendste? Jugend Sport *32:* 377 (1975).
52 Pilz, G.A.: Verhalten beim Skifahren. Sportarzt Sportmed. *2:* 66–103 (1977).
53 Potter, H.: Sicher Sporttreiben, pp. 76–77 (SUVA und Winterthur-Versicherungen, Switzerland 1982).
54 Pöschl, M.; Krieger, G.: Todesfälle beim Sport und medizinische Fragen ihrer Prophylaxe. Münch. med. Wschr. *105:* 2205–2216 (1963).
55 Riddell, J.: The ski runs of Switzerland (Michael Joseph, London 1957).
56 Rigos, F.J.; Gross, K.E.: Ski injuries. J. Am. med. Ass. *166:* 972 (1958).
57 Röthlisberger, M.F.; Herwig, O.K.: Art und Häufigkeit von Skiunfällen in Arosa. Praxis *65:* 346 (1976).
58 Scharfetter, F.: Schädel-Hirn-Traumen durch Skiunfälle. Med. Sport *2:* 40 (1976).
59 Sellier, K.: Das Schädel-Hirn-Trauma. Z. Rechtsmed. *68:* 239–252 (1971).
60 Schneider, R.C.: Head and neck injuries in football, pp. 216–277 (Williams & Wilkins, Baltimore 1973).
61 Ski Atlas 1983: DSV-Tips für Schleppliftfahrer, p. 716 (1983).
62 Stoffel, H.P.: Studien zur Geschichte der russischen Skisportterminologie. Slacica helv. *1975:* 34–43.
63 Subczynski, J.A.: One stage debridement and plastic repair of compound comminuted depressed skull fracture with methylmethacrylate. J. Trauma *17:* 467–469 (1977).
64 Terbizan, N.: Eine Statistik der Skiverletzungen. Wschr. Unfallheilk. *7:* 337 (1966).
65 Vanderfield, G.: The problems of head injuries in sport. Bull post-grad. comm. med. Univ. Syndey *30:* 122–126 (1974).
66 Youmans, J.R.: Skull fracture and management of open head injury. Neurol. Surg. *2:* 969–977 (1973).

Subject Index